NUTRITION AND DIET RESEARCH PROGRESS

FOLIC ACID

PROPERTIES, MEDICAL USES AND HEALTH BENEFITS

Nutrition and Diet Research Progress

Additional books in this series can be found on Nova's website under the Series tab.

Additional E-books in this series can be found on Nova's website under the E-book tab.

NUTRITION AND DIET RESEARCH PROGRESS

FOLIC ACID

PROPERTIES, MEDICAL USES AND HEALTH BENEFITS

MÁRIA SZABÓ
AND
EVE VARGA
EDITORS

Nova Science Publishers, Inc.
New York

For permission to use material from this book please contact us:
Telephone 631-231-7269; Fax 631-231-8175
Web Site: http://www.novapublishers.com

LIBRARY OF CONGRESS CATALOGING-IN-PUBLICATION DATA

Folic acid : properties, medical uses, and health benefits / editors, Maria Szabs and Eve Varga.
p. ; cm.
Includes bibliographical references and index.
ISBN 978-1-62100-867-5 (hardcover)
I. Szabs, Maria, M.D. II. Varga, Eve.
[DNLM: 1. Folic Acid--therapeutic use. 2. Folic Acid--pharmacology. 3. Health Education. 4. Neural Tube Defects--prevention & control. QU 188]

615.3--dc23

2011038602

Published by Nova Science Publishers, Inc. † New York

Contents

Preface

Folic acid is one of 13 essential vitamins that can be obtained from dietary sources or supplements. Despite a relative abundance of folic acid in food, its deficiency is frequent and can arise as a consequence of poor diet, chronic illness, drugs, and malabsorption. Folic acid is essential for the functioning of the nervous system. In this new book, the authors present topical research in the study of the properties, medical uses and health benefits of folic acid including the role of folic acid in psychiatric disorders; the importance of folic acid in fertility, miscarriage and preterm birth; the actions of folic acid in the prevention of neural tube defects; folic acid and prostate cancer; photobiological properties of folic acid and how folic acid and B12 supplementation improves the survival of elderly hemodialysis patients.

Chapter 1 - Among structural birth defects, i.e. congenital abnormalities, neural-tube defects are the common and severe congenital abnormalities of nervous system. Recent intervention trials showed that about 90% of neural-tube defects are preventable by periconception (at least one month before conception and at least two months after conception) folic acid-containing multivitamin, while about 70 % by periconception folic acid supplementation. In addition this method is appropriate to reduce the birth prevalence of cardiovascular malformations, the most common congenital abnormalities. These findings theoretically resulted in a breakthrough in the prevention of congenital abnormalities; nevertheless this method is not used frequently in medical practice. The four possible uses of periconception folic acid/multivitamin supplementation are presented: (i) dietary intake, but alone folate rich diet is not appropriate for the prevention of neural-tube defects and other congenital abnormalities; (ii) periconception folic acid/multivitamin supplementation, however, women with unplanned pregnancies cannot utilize this simple and cheap method because it needs the onset of folic acid/multivitamin use at least 1-3 months before conception; (iii) flour fortification with folic acid, but it is not used in Europe and (iv) the recent attempt for the use of combination of oral contraceptives with 6S-5-methyltetrahydrofolate ("folate") as a compromise because of the missed opportunities mentioned above. Recent studies have shown that folic acid, particularly during the third trimester can also reduce the rate of preterm births. In conclusion folic acid is able to reduce the occurrence of congenital abnormalities and preterm births, the two major factors of infant mortality and handicaps.

Chapter 2 - Folic acid is one of 13 essential vitamins that can be obtained from dietary sources or supplements. Despite a relative abundance of folic acid in food, its deficiency is frequent and can arise as a consequence of poor diet, chronic illness, drugs, malabsorption, and an increased demand. Noteworthy, folic acid is essential for the functioning of the nervous system, since it plays an important role in neuroplasticity and in the maintenance of neuronal integrity. Several studies have indicated that folic acid plays a role in the pathophysiology and/or treatment of neuropsychiatric disorders such as depression, bipolar disorder, and schizophrenia. Individuals with low blood levels of folic acid seem more prone to the development of these neuropsychiatric disorders. Moreover, this vitamin deficiency has been correlated with a reduced effectiveness or a poor response to medication such as antidepressants. Although several preclinical and clinical studies have indicated a link between folic acid deficiency and neuropsychiatric disorders, the mechanisms underlying the beneficial effects of folic acid against these diseases have not been fully elucidated. This chapter presents an overview of the preclinical and clinical studies that have pointed to the link between folic acid and psychiatric disorders highlighting the evidence for the use of folic acid supplementation as a potential therapeutic strategy for the treatment of these diseases.

Chapter 3 - Folic acid is an essential micronutrient, and deficiency is linked to an increased risk of neural tube defects in the developing embryo. Knowing the importance of folic acid during embryogenesis, the authors sought to examine its effects on other aspects of reproduction including fertility, preterm birth, and miscarriage. Studies indicate that folic acid supplementation aids in spermatogenesis. In female reproduction, low homocysteine levels are associated with improved oocyte quality and maturity, as well as increased efficacy of IVF treatments. After evaluating maternal serum folate status and periconceptual folic acid supplementation, researchers found an association between increased folic acid and a reduced risk of preterm birth. However, studies have presented conflicting findings on the role of folic acid in prevention of miscarriage, with some proposing a protective effect of folic acid on the developing fetus. With promising data suggesting that folic acid plays a major role in reproduction outside the realm of neural tube development, more research is needed to clarify the extent of the impact of folic acid supplementation and the mechanism underlying its benefit. Further, supplementation has the potential to reduce healthcare costs associated with these reproductive issues.

Chapter 4 - The relationship between folic acid (FA) and neural tube defects (NTDs) has been well documented in the last twenty years. Increased FA intake due to fortification methods have been shown to reduce the incidence of NTDs significantly. While FA's role as a methylating agent has been established, the processes behind the development of NTDs are still being studied. Several proposed mechanisms involving metabolic deficiencies of factors of the remethylation cycle have demonstrated exaggerated behaviors in diseased states. Diabetes mellitus contributes to a higher incidence of NTDs, which can be ameliorated by FA supplementation. Hyperglycemia appears to adversely affect proliferation and normal apoptosis of neural progenitor cells, as well as placental uptake of FA, through mechanisms of oxidative stress. Similar attenuation is seen in the treatment of women with epilepsy. The interaction of FA and antiepileptic drugs (AEDs) presents a complication in the care of pregnancy. AEDs are associated with increased rates of NTDs, thus making prenatal planning imperative. This includes periconceptual FA fortification, administration of the lowest possible dose of AEDs, and antenatal screening for NTDs. Current research supports increased intake of FA in women, especially those in a diseased state. Further research is necessary in order to ascertain the true limits of FA action.

Chapter 5 - In a concerted effort, a statewide coalition educated women of childbearing age about the relationship between folic acid consumption and the risk of neural tube birth defects (NTDs) among infants. Whether a pregnancy is planned or unplanned, research indicates that timely folic acid intake among women can reduce the risk of having an NTD-affected pregnancy. According to the Centers for Disease Control and Prevention (CDC), consumption of folic acid, a B vitamin, may reduce a woman's NTD-risk by up to 70% if the vitamin is taken 30 days prior to conception and every day throughout pregnancy. The United States Public Health Service (USPHS) recommends that women of childbearing age consume 400 micrograms of folic acid every day and notes that special situations may require higher intake levels.

A university extension service and a Folic Acid/Health Pregnancy Task Force formed a strategic statewide coalition to promote the "Folic Acid Every Day" message through media, classes, and health fairs using CDC- and locally-developed resources. The message was promoted by more than 131 coalition partners including: the National Folic Acid Council, a medical foundation, the state chapter of the March of Dimes, Extension agents, regional Women, Infants and Children (WIC) staff, Public Health staff, commodity groups, franchise restaurants, and pharmacies. Using feedback from task force members, a communication-based intervention campaign was developed and modeled after the CDC's *Ready or Not* campaign. Coalition members administered a baseline survey (n=422), conducted a folic-acid education intervention, and administered a second survey (n=349) following the intervention.

Thousands of people were reached with folic acid information through the use of mass media advertising including radio public service announcements, bathroom stall ads, a statewide radio program, and newspaper columns. The folic acid message was promoted through newspaper columns, e-mail blasts, press releases, and a Web site. Additionally, the coalition promoted and distributed the folic acid message on a variety of materials including recipe cards, educational DVDs, brochures, posters, congratulations cards provided with marriage licenses, oral contraceptive packet auxiliary labels, and restaurant and grocery store coupons.

Following the intervention, folic acid awareness, knowledge, and supplement intake behavior increased among women of childbearing age. About 76% of the survey participants were aware of folic acid (up 1% from Survey One; $p > .05$), 65% were able to identify folic acid as a B vitamin (up 12% from Survey One; $p < .05$), 79% recognized the association between folic acid and NTDs (up 10% from Survey One; $p < .05$), and 45% were aware of the daily folic acid intake recommendation of 400 mcg (up 18% from Survey One; $p < .05$). Approximately 46% of the participants were able to identify that women of childbearing age should take folic acid prior to and during pregnancy (up 14% from Survey One; $p < .05$), and 58% of the participants were taking folic acid every day (up 17% from Survey One; $p < .05$). The follow-up survey results indicated that task force members raised folic acid awareness and knowledge among women within 63% of the state's counties, including the most populous cities. In conclusion, an effective folic acid education campaign may serve to reduce the number of females at risk for having an NTD-affected pregnancy during childbearing age, and this project may serve as a model for other state coalitions.

Chapter 6 - Increasing evidence continues to indicate that dietary nutrients can significantly influence the incidence of many cancer types. One dietary component that has been implicated as a crucial factor in carcinogenesis is folate. Folate is a water-soluble member of the vitamin B group that plays a key role in DNA methylation, synthesis, and repair. The synthetic form of folate is folic acid, and this form is more biologically available than the natural folate form. While several epidemiological studies suggest that higher folate intake corresponds with decreased risk of many human malignancies, data showing the relationship between folate intake and the risk of prostate cancer are limited and inconsistent. Importantly, a clear demonstration of the benefits of dietary folate for reducing prostate cancer risk is yet to be established. With recent biotechnological capabilities to genetically engineer crops to have increased availability of important biological nutrients, future clinical studies directed at investigating the correlation between folate and chemoprevention of prostate cancer will be challenging but important, coming with the promise to yield high public health benefits.

Chapter 7 - Folic acid is an important human nutrient. This compound consists of *p*-aminobenzoyl-L-glutamic acid and pteridine, which absorb ultraviolet A (UVA) light. UVA-irradiation to folic acid results in the decomposition and the formation of unconjugated pteridines through intra-molecular electron transfer and subsequent reactions. The formed pteridines act as strong photosensitizer to damage DNA via electron transfer from guanines, leading to the formation of various oxidized products, including 8-oxo-7,8-dihydro-2'-deoxyguanine, a main indicator of oxidative DNA damage. These findings suggest that photolysis of folic acid may contribute to skin cancer by solar UVA radiation. The conjugation of the pteridine and the aminobenzoyl moiety in folic acid structure may play an important role in the prevention of UVA carcinogesis. On the other hand, fluorescence intensity of folic acid, which scarcely fluoresces, is markedly enhanced by reactive oxygen species through oxidative decomposition. This character can be applied for the fluorometry of hydrogen peroxide and the determination of singlet oxygen quantum yields of various photosensitizers.

Chapter 8 - A large part of hemodialysis patients is over 65 years old. They often have vitamin B deficiency, hyperhomocysteinemia and high mortality rate. Recent meta-analysis have shown a significant decrease of cardiovascular disease in hyperhomocysteinemic end-stage renal disease patients treated with folic acid, but until now there are no data about the long-term effect of folic acid plus vitamin B12 on survival rate.

A long-term observational analysis was performed to assess the effects of vitamin B therapy on survival rate of incident hemodialysis patient over 65 years old. A large part of hemodialysis patients derived from previous prospective studies analysing the effects of folic acid on cardiovascular morbidity. 189 patients started haemodialysis, but only 141 patients had a follow-up time larger than 3 months. The mean age was 76 ± 0,5 years (65-86). The mean follow-up time was 959 ± 66 days (99-3518). 106 of 141 (75%) patients died. The median survival time was 2,7 years (0,3-9,6). Patients were sorted in two groups derived from folic acid and vitamin B12 treatment: group A (98 patients without vitamin B therapy or folic acid alone) and group B (43 patients with double vitamin B therapy). The median survival time was significantly different in the two groups: respectively equal to 1,8 years in group A and 3,9 years in group B ($p< 0,01$). Univariate regression analysis showed that death was directly dependent by age (χ^2: 8,2 ; $p< 0,01$), presence of central venous catheter at starting hemodialysis (χ^2: 10 – $p< 0,01$), late referral to our care (χ^2: 7 ; $p< 0,01$), and inversely related to double therapy with folic acid and vitamin B12 (χ^2: 18 ; $p< 0,0001$). Logistic multiple regression analysis demonstrated a strong reverse association between double vitamin B therapy and mortality (Coef/SE: -4,0 ; χ^2: 25,1 ; p value: <0,001).

Folic acid and vitamin B12 therapy was inversely associated with mortality in elderly hemodialysis patients. Homocysteine-lowering therapy may be useful to reduce cardiovascular and bone morbidity. Homocysteine-lowering effect may be reached with combination treatment using multivitamin B therapy, N-acetylcysteine and mixed dialysis therapies as high flux bicarbonate dialysis, internal hemodiafiltration, hemodiafiltration with endogenous reinfusion and on-line hemodiafiltration. Nowadays, it is important to perform a well-designed randomized controlled trial analyzing the effects of homocysteine-lowering therapies on hard end-points.

In: Folic Acid
Editors: Mária Szabó and Eve Varga
ISBN: 978-1-62100-867-5

Chapter I

Folic Acid and Pregnancy: Properties, Medical Uses and Health Benefits

Andrew E. Czeizel[1,*], István Dudás[1], Attila Vereczkey[2] and Ferenc Bánhidy[3]

[1]Foundation for the Community Control of Hereditary Diseases, Budapest
[2]Periconception Care Unit, Human Reproduction Institute, Budapest
[3]Second Department of Obstetrics and Gynecology, Semmelweis University, School of Medicine, Budapest, Hungary

To the memory of Professor Tom K. A. B. ESKES (1933-2011), excellent gynaecologist/obstetrician, founder of a great scientific team in University Hospital Nijmegen, the Netherland and a good friend

* Correspondence: Andrew E. Czeizel, Hungary, 1026 Budapest, Törökvész lejtõ 32. E-mail: czeizel@interware.hu.

Abstract

Among structural birth defects, i.e. congenital abnormalities, neural-tube defects are the common and severe congenital abnormalities of nervous system. Recent intervention trials showed that about 90% of neural-tube defects are preventable by periconception (at least one month before conception and at least two months after conception) folic acid-containing multivitamin, while about 70 % by periconception folic acid supplementation. In addition this method is appropriate to reduce the birth prevalence of cardiovascular malformations, the most common congenital abnormalities. These findings theoretically resulted in a breakthrough in the prevention of congenital abnormalities; nevertheless this method is not used frequently in medical practice. The four possible uses of periconception folic acid/multivitamin supplementation are presented: (i) dietary intake, but alone folate rich diet is not appropriate for the prevention of neural-tube defects and other congenital abnormalities; (ii) periconception folic acid/multivitamin supplementation, however, women with unplanned pregnancies cannot utilize this simple and cheap method because it needs the onset of folic acid/multivitamin use at least 1-3 months before conception; (iii) flour fortification with folic acid, but it is not used in Europe and (iv) the recent attempt for the use of combination of oral contraceptives with 6S-5-methyltetrahydrofolate ("folate") as a compromise because of the missed opportunities mentioned above. Recent studies have shown that folic acid, particularly during the third trimester can also reduce the rate of preterm births. In conclusion folic acid is able to reduce the occurrence of congenital abnormalities and preterm births, the two major factors of infant mortality and handicaps.

Keywords: Neural-tube defects, cardiovascular malformations, folic acid, multivitamins, preterm births, prevention.

Vitamins are organic molecules which in small amounts are obligatory nutrients, because in general they cannot be synthesized de novo in human beings. (Only vitamin D can be manufactured by the body at a sufficient rate.) At present 13 chemicals, or groups of chemicals are classified as vitamins. The group of water soluble B vitamins consists of 8 vitamins, and one of them, vitamin B11 or B9 (folate/folic acid) recently has resulted in a breakthrough in the prevention of structural birth defects, i.e. *congenital abnormalities (CAs).*

Folate and Folic Acid

The natural monoglutamate folate was discovered by Lucy Wills 80 years ago (Wills, 1931) and she recommended using the term vitamin B11 as a "twin" of vitamin B12. Later the polyglutamate form of this vitamin, as *folic acid (FA)* was produced (Hoffbrand, 1965). Humans cannot produce folate, the major dietary sources of folates are fresh and frozen green leafy vegetables, citrus fruits and juices, liver, wheat bread and legumes, such as beans. Thus the requirement of this water-soluble vitamin is supplied partly by the dietary intakes of folates, partly by the use of synthetic FA, and at the estimation of necessary dose we have to add these two forms of vitamin B11 (though this vitamin is named as vitamin B9 in France and some other countries).

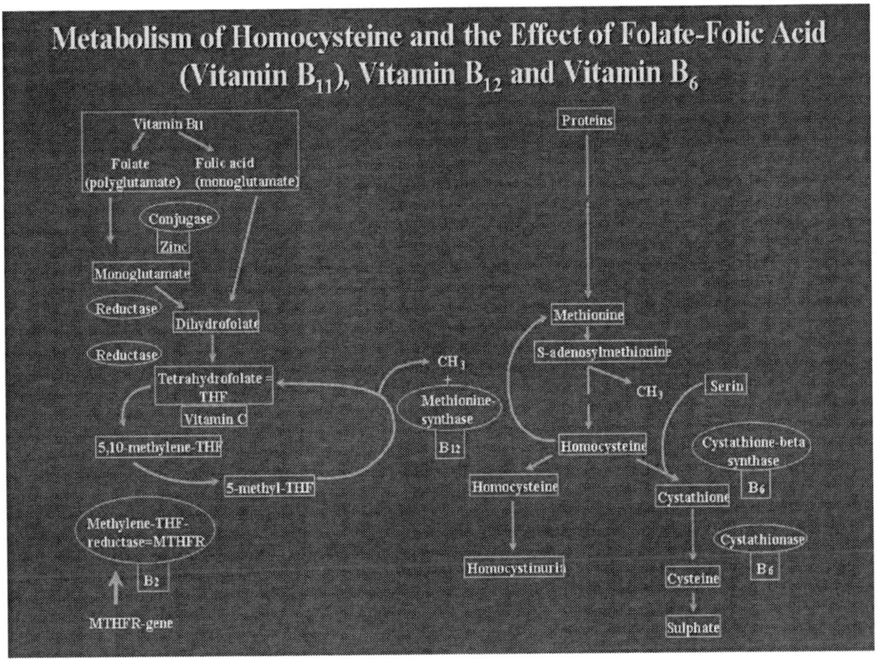

Figure 1. THF = tetrahydrofolate, MTHFR = methylenetetrahydrofolate-reductase, CH_3 = methyl group.

After dietary intake of monoglutamate folates and intended supply of synthetic polyglutamate FA (Figure), these two forms of this vitamin have absorption in the cells of the upper small intestine. FA can absorb directly while folate is changed into monoglutamate form by conjugase enzyme. In the next step these monoglutamates are converted to dihydrofolate and then to *tetrahydrofolate (THF)* by reductase enzymes. THF is the parent compound of all biological active forms of this vitamin. THF is converted to 5,10-methylene-THF and *5-methylene-THF (5-MTHF)* before transfer into the hepatic portal vein which then leads to the liver and onwards to the systematic blood circulation and all body tissues.

The above metabolites of folate can transfer rapidly from maternal organism to the placenta, though the placenta stores folates and their transfer occur only after placental tissue vitamin receptors are saturated (Landon et at, 1975, Baker et al., 1981). Folate deficiency is common during pregnancy if diet is not supplemented with folic acid, because maternal serum/plasma and red cell blood folate level decline during pregnancy (Chanarin et al., 1968, Ek et al., 1981) due to decreased absorption, accelerated breakdown of folates, increased urinary loss and last but not least fetal transfer. The most common complication of maternal folate deficiency is megaloblastic anemia (Chanarin et al., 1959).

Folates are required for cell division and cell maintenance, because it acts as a co-enzyme in the transfer and processing of one-carbon units and plays an important role in nucleotide (thymidine) synthesis which is essential for the *de novo* construction or repair of DNA. In addition this vitamin as a coenzyme is needed for protein synthesis, among others hemoglobin thus is important in hematopoiesis. Folates are also key factors in the "site-specific" methylation of the cytosine base in DNA, which regulates gene expression. Finally another major function of folates is the re-methylation of plasma homocysteine to methionine, only this function will be shown later.

Previously there were two forms of FA as medicinal products: tablets of FA and FA-containing multivitamins for oral intake. In the recent years, a nature-identical folate of 5-MTHF as 6S-5-MTHF has been synthesized as a calcium salt and marketed as Metafolin[R] (Wright et al., 2010). Thus it is a synthetic product but equal with its natural form, thus the term folate is correct. The possible benefits of 6S-5-MTHF use compared to FA supplementation was summarized previously (Czeizel at al., 2011).

History of Prevention of Neural-Tube Defects by Folic Acid or Multivitamins

Among CAs of the central nervous system, the group of *neural-tube defects (NTD)* is the most frequent and the most tragic CAs.

First Hibbard (1964) reported a higher rate of CAs (3%) in the infants of folate-deficient mothers than in controls (1.6%). Later Hibbard and Smithells (1965) showed a relationship between human embryopathy and a deficiency of folate metabolism. Finally Smithells et al (1976) focused their studies on NTD and demonstrated the role of vitamin deficiencies in the origin of this CA-group.

The brain and spinal cord develop from the neural-tube which is formed by dorsal folding of the neural plate after 15th postconception day. The fusion of this folding proceeds in cranial and caudal directions and is normally complete in humans at 21 to 26 postconception days in the cranial pole and 23 to 28 days in the caudal pole, respectively (Czeizel, 2008), therefore these periods correspond to the critical period of anencephaly and spina bifida. However, it is necessary to consider that at present the so-called gestational age is calculated from the first day of the last menstrual period in clinical practice, therefore it is necessary to add 14 days to the postconception/fetal age to estimate the gestational age. Thus the critical period of anencephaly is between 35th and 40th gestational days, while spina bifida had this period between 37th and 42nd gestational days.

Anencephaly is virtual absence of the forebrain and the skull vault caused by failure of closure on the cranial neuropore of the neural-tube. Spina bifida is the closure defect of the caudal end of the neural-tube therefore the clinical manifestation is a midline defect of the osseous spine usually affecting the posterior arches. Occipital encephalocele is part of the NTD-spectrum but with different pathogenesis (Czeizel, 2010), therefore this type of NTD is not discussed here.

At the evaluation of NTD cases the first task is to differentiate the so-called isolated and multiple-syndromic cases. The definition of isolated CA is only one organ is affected while syndromic CAs have concurrence of two or more CAs in the same person affecting at least two different organ systems. However, isolated CAs may be manifested as seemingly multiple CA, e.g. spina bifida sequence, because the primary defect spina bifida frequently associated with secondary clubfoot, hydrocephalus, etc.

At present the etiology of NTD is not known exactly but most *isolated NTD* cases have multifactorial origin, i.e. polygenic predisposition with an interaction by external agents which can trigger or suppress this genetic predisposition. The polygenic predisposition is confirmed by the recurrence risk that is 10-folds higher in the first degree relatives (mainly sibs) of patients with NTD than the first occurrence of NTD in a given population. On the other hand, the importance of environmental agents is indicated by the socio-economic dependence of NTD (the occurrence of NTD is much lower in the highest class than in the lowest class) and their obvious populations differences (0.2-10.5 per 1000) in different geographical regions, and last but not least by the preventive effect of FA. Syndromic NTD cases are caused by chromosomal aberrations (e.g. trisomy 13), mutant major genes (e.g. Meckel-Gruber syndrome with autosomal recessive inheritance) and teratogens (e.g. antiepileptic valprote). However, it is worth mentioning that syndromic NTD cases represent only a minor part of all NTD cases (less than 10%), thus the isolated manifestation is characteristic for NTD.

Anencephaly is lethal, while the life expectancy of patients with spina bifida has improved significantly due to the early surgical intervention but survivors have multiple handicaps.

The occurrence of NTD depends on maternal socio-economic status (Elwood et al., 1992), as it was mentioned previously, thus R. W. Smithells hypothesized that undernutrition could be the common factor in the origin of NTD. His group tested therefore the effect of diet supplemented with a multivitamin containing 0.36 mg FA in the first intervention trial (Smithells et al., 1980). Women who had had one or more previous infants with NTD were supplemented by this multivitamin during the periconception period while controls were recruited among similar women who were already pregnant without vitamin supplementation. The results of this intervention study were published separately for the Yorkshire region of the UK (Smithells et al., 1989) and Northern Ireland (Nevin and Seller, 1990), and they found *91% and 83% reduction in NTD recurrence*, respectively.

However, the results of Smithells' study were not accepted by some experts because of possible selection bias. They supposed that more educated and well-to-do females with a lower risk for NTD had a higher participation in the multivitamin supplemented group. Thus a *randomized controlled trial* (RCT) was organized by the Medical Research Council (MRC) of the UK in 7 countries (43% of participants came from Hungary). There were four supplementation groups: FA (4 mg), other vitamins, FA + other vitamins and minerals as control. The MRC Vitamin Study found that a *pharmacological dose (4 mg) of FA alone can reduce NTD recurrence by 71%,* (0.8% vs. 4.3%; RR with 95% CI: 0.29, 0.12-0.71) (MRC Vitamin Study, 1991).

The periconception multivitamin supplementation was incorporated into the *Hungarian Periconception Service* (HPS) launched in 1984 (Czeizel, 1999) as a RCT. Half of participants were supplied by a micronutrient combination (the so-called 'multivitamin' containing 12 vitamins, 4 minerals, and 3 trace elements) (Table 1), while the other half of participants were not supplied by this multivitamin randomly. These women were supplemented at least during one month before conception and at least during two months after conception, i.e. in periconception period.

There were two major questions of the Hungarian RCT following the publications of the above two 'recurrence' studies: (I) "Does folic acid-containing multivitamin reduce the risk of *first* occurrence of NTD?" About 95% of women who have fetus or infants with isolated NTD had no previous NTD pregnancies, thus the prevention of their first occurrence would be a real public health success. (II) The pharmacological dose (4 mg) of FA used in MRC Vitamin Study may have some adverse effects, thus it was necessary to evaluate the *physiological dose* (1 mg or less) of FA. Thus the efficacy of a multivitamin containing 0.8 mg FA was tested.

NTD did not occur in 2,471 offspring of the multivitamin group, while 6 NTD were found in 2,391 offspring of no-multivitamin group (p=0.01; RR with 95% CI: 0.07, 0.01-0.13). Thus, the Hungarian RCT demonstrated first that a multivitamin containing 0.8 mg FA prevented *about 90% of the first occurrences of NTD* (Czeizel and Dudás, 1992).

The unexpected finding of the Hungarian RCT was a significant reduction in the total rate of major CAs: 20.6 per 1000 in the multivitamin and 40.6 per 1000 in the no-multivitamin group (RR with 95% CI: 0.53, 0.35–0.70). The detailed analysis of data based on the personal medical examination in all children indicated a significant reduction in urinary tract's CAs (RR with 95% CI: 0.21, 0.05-0.95) and cardiovascular CAs (RR with 95% CI: 0.42, 0.19-0.98). There was also some but not significant reduction in the rate of congenital limb deficiencies (RR with 95% CI: 0.19, 0.03-1.18) and pyloric stenosis (RR with 95% CI: 0.24, 0.05-1.14) in the multivitamin group.

After the exclusion 6 NTD cases, the difference in the rate of major CAs between the two study-groups remained very highly significant (p<0.0001). In conclusion, periconceptional multivitamin supplementation reduced not only the occurrence of NTD but also the rate of some other major CAs (Czeizel, 1993b, 1996, 1988).

For ethical reasons, the Hungarian RCT could not be continued, thus a *cohort controlled trial (CCT)* was designed to collect more data regarding the preventive effect of this multivitamin for NTD and other CAs (Czeizel et al., 2004). All participants in the HPS were supplied with the multivitamin used in RCT while women for unsupplemented cohort were recruited at the 14th week of pregnancy without vitamin use from the regional prenatal care clinics and they were matched to each pregnant woman of the supplemented cohort. The protective effect of this multivitamin for the *reduction of NTD* was confirmed in these 3,056 "pairs" (1 vs. 9; OR with 95% CI: 0.11, 0.01-0.91).

Table 1. Composition of different vitamins, minerals and trace elements in the tested folic acid-containing multivitamin (i.e. micronutrient combination)

Elevit Pronatal®	
Components Doses	
Vitamins	
A	1000 IU
B_1	1.6 mg
B_2	1.8 mg
Nicotinamid	19.0 mg
B_6	2.6 mg
Calcium pantothenate	10.0 mg
Biotin	0.2 mg
B_{12}	4.0 mg
C	100.0 mg
D	500.0 IU
E	15.0 mg
Folic acid	0.8 mg
Minerals	
Calcium	125.0 mg
Phosphorus	125.0 mg
Magnesium	100.0 mg
Iron	60.0 mg
Trace elements	
Copper	1.0 mg
Manganese	1.0 mg
Zinc	7.5 mg

However, the total prevalence of cases with syndromic NTD was not reduced either in the RCT or in the CCT (Czeizel and Medveczki, 2003). Later the population based Hungarian Case-Control Surveillance of Congenital Abnormalities (Czeizel et al., 2001) was also appropriate to compare the rate of multiple CAs including syndromic NTDs in the offspring of pregnant women with or without FA/multivitamin supplementation, and there was no difference between these two study-groups (Czeizel et al., 2006). Thus syndromic NTD is not preventable by FA or FA-containing multivitamins.

Later the results of only one intervention trial was reported, the efficacy of 0.4 mg FA for the prevention of first occurrence of NTD was shown in a *Chinese-US study* (Berry et al., 1999). There was 79% reduction in the risk of NTD in areas with high rates of NTD (6.5 per 1000), while this reduction was 41% in areas with low rates of NTD (0.8 per 1000).

Many observational studies of FA-containing multivitamins or FA alone were also published, which confirmed the prevention of NTD, but above only the data of intervention trials were summarised.

In conclusion FA (0.4-4.0 mg) can prevent 40-70%, while FA-containing multivitamins about 90 % of NTD if these medicinal products were used during the periconception period.

Prevention of other Congenital Abnormalities

The Hungarian RCT showed the efficacy of a multivitamin in the reduction of some other CAs, mainly *cardiovascular CAs (CCAs)* as well. Thus the major aim of the Hungarian CCT was to confirm or reject these unexpected findings.

In the Hungarian CCT the rate of CAs was again significantly reduced (OR with 95% CI: 0.74, 0.58-0.94), explained mainly by the lower occurrence of CCAs (OR with 95% CI: 0.60, 0.38-0.96). In the group of CCAs, particularly ventricular septal defect showed a very significant reduction (OR with 95% CI: 0.26, 0.09–0.72) in the supplemented cohort. Some observational studies also showed significant reduction in the birth prevalence of CCAs particularly conotruncal CAs after the use of FA-containing multivitamins (Botto et al., 1996, Botto et al., 2000).

CCAs are most common among major CAs and nearly half of CA-related infant mortality is caused by CCAs. Among 1000 live-births, 7–8 were affected with CCA in different studies. In a Hungarian population-based study of 2,259 children based on the pediatric cardiologic examination and/or autopsy report of each individual child resulted in 10.2 per 1000 birth prevalence of CCA (Mészáros et al., 1975). The total (birth + fetal) prevalence of NTD was 2.8 per 1000 in Hungary (Czeizel and Révész, 1970), thus the ratio of CCAs:NTD is 3.6:1.0. In many countries (e.g. USA) the rate of NTD is lower, thus CCA:NTD ratio is higher.

The two Hungarian intervention trials indicated about 40% reduction in risk for CCAs after FA-containing multivitamin supplementation. The protective effect of high doses (about 6 mg) FA alone was also found for CCAs in the Hungarian Case-Control Surveillance of Congenital Abnormalities (Czeizel et al, 1996c). The meta-analysis of both case-control studies (OR with 95% CI: 0.78, 0.67–0.92) and cohort studies or RCT (OR with 95% CI: 0.61, 0.40–0.92) indicated a reduction in the risk of CCAs (Goh et al., 2006). The significant 6% reduction (OR with 95% CI: 0.94, 0.90–0.97) was found in the prevalence of severe CCAs in Quebec, Canada, after FA fortification of grain products (Ionescu-Ittu et al., 2009). In addition a registry-based case-control study also showed the protective effect of periconception FA or FA-containing multivitamin use for all types of CCAs (OR with CI: 0.82, 0.68–0.98), particularly of isolated septal defects (0.62, 0.47–0.82) (van Beynum et al., 2010).

The reduction of CCAs by this new preventive method has a similar great public health importance as the prevention of NTD. As we mentioned previously, we calculate about a 90 % reduction after the periconceptional FA-containing multivitamin supplementation (thus the total rate of NTD is reduced from 2.8 to 0.3 per 1000), while this reduction is about 40 % in CCAs, thus the total rate of 10.2 is reduced to 6.1 per 1000. However, if we estimate the reduction of these two CAs in absolute numbers per 100,000 pregnancies/births, this preventive method can result in reduction of 408 cases with CCA and 252 cases with NTD.

Nevertheless, whereas the prevention of NTD by FA and FA-containing multivitamins was accepted with enthusiasm in the international scientific community in the early 1990s and prompted new recommendations for their practical implementation, the new data regarding the prevention of CCAs have been received with reservation and without any further recommendation. Partly, it is understandable because different CAs have different origin, therefore difficult to believe that such a simple vitamin supplementation can reduce some different CAs. It is necessary therefore to clearly identify the mechanism of periconception FA/multivitamin use in the reduction of specific

CAs. On the contrary, the possible prevention of CCAs was confirmed in several studies, thus it would be necessary to include the prevention of CCAs with high prevalence worldwide into the public health action and information for prospective mothers.

In the Hungarian CCT, the CAs of urinary tract did not show significant difference between supplemented and unsupplemented cohort (OR with 95% CI: 0.71, 0.33-1.50), though stenosis of pelvicureteric junction (2 vs. 13) had a reduction (OR with 95% CI: 0.19, 0.04–0.86). Li et al. (1995) and Werler et al.(1999) also found a significant reduction in the rate of urinary tract's CAs after multivitamin use in the first trimester of pregnancy.

The rate of limb deficiencies (OR with 95% CI: 0.33, 0.01-3.71) and pyloric stenosis (OR with 95% CI: 0.0. 0.0-26.8) showed again a decreasing trend in the supplemented cohort in the Hungarian CCT. One observational US study found a significant reduction of congenital limb deficiencies after multivitamin supplementation (Yang et al., 1997).

Finally it is worth mentioning that there was no reduction in the rate of isolated orofacial cleft (cleft lip with or without cleft palate: CL ± CP and cleft palate only) either in the Hungarian RCT (RR with 95% CI: 0.8, 0.2-2.7) or in the Hungarian CCT (OR with 95% CI: 1.6, 0.3-2.9). Previously Tolarova (1982) reported a protective effect of a multivitamin and FA (10 mg) during the periconception period for the recurrence of cleft lips. On the other hand, 30% reduction was found in the occurrence of CL ± CP in the Hungarian Case-Control Surveillance of Congenital Abnormalities after the use of high dose (in general 6 mg) of FA alone (Czeizel et al.,1999), thus a dose-dependent preventive effect of FA for CL ± CP cannot be excluded.

In conclusion, several observational studies confirmed the result of the Hungarian intervention trials that FA-containing multivitamin supplementation is appropriate for the prevention of other CAs beyond NTD as well and it is extremely important from public health aspect because NTD represents only 3-12% of all major CAs. FA or FA-containing multivitamin supplementation offers a breakthrough in the prevention of NTD and some other CAs because can reduce about one third of CAs (Tarusco, 2004) and provide a better alternative than the elective termination of pregnancy after the diagnosis of severe fetal defects.

The Possible Role of Hyperhomocysteinemia in the Origin of Certain Congenital Abnormalities

The origin of NTD can be explained by gene-environmental (such as dietary deficiency) interaction. Several genes and environmental factors contribute to the origin of NTD, here only one – the most established – hyperhomocysteinemia (Bolander-Gouaille, 2002) is summarised because hyperhomocysteinemia plays a role in the origin of at least some part of NTD.

When meat, fish or plant proteins are digested, amino acids, among others, methionine, are released, and methionine is converted to homocysteine (Figure). Homocysteine is a toxic metabolite; therefore humans neutralize it normally as soon as possible. On the one hand, homocysteine is metabolized via the transsulfuration pathway to form cystathionine catalyzed by cystathionine β-synthase and serine hydroxymethyltransferase. The latter enzymes require pyridoxal 5'-phosphate, i.e. vitamin B6 as a cofactor. On the other hand, remethylation of homocysteine to methionine is catalyzed by methionine-synthase. This enzyme requires vitamin B12 as a cofactor and 5-MTHF as the methyl donor. The latter explains the importance of *folate-FA deficiency* in the origin of NTD.

The most important cause of hyperhomocysteinemia and/or lack of methionine are the polymorphism of *MTHF-reductase (MTHFR) gene* (Goyette et al., 1994). A 677C→T mutation has been identified in the *MTHFR*-gene and it results in thermolabile variant (Ala225Val) of *MTHFR-enzyme* with 40% reduction in its activity of CT (heterozygote) and with very low (about 70% reduction) activity of TT (homozygote) forms (Frosst et al., 1995). Vitamin B2 is a cofactor of MTHFR-enzyme. The enzyme variants due to its mutant gene-pairs cannot effectively catalyze the pathway of 5,10-methylene-THF to 5-MTHF, i.e., the methyl donor for methionine-synthase. About 10-12 % of the European population is homozygous (TT) while about 40% are heterozygotes (CT) for this polymorphism of MTHFR-gene pairs. The frequency of TT and CT genotypes is 11.1% and 45.2%, respectively, in the Hungarian population (Wilcken et al., 2003).

The lower activity of MTHFR-enzyme reduces the production of 5-MTHR and increases plasma homocysteine level which causes a delay in the closure of neural-tube, thus indirectly NTD. If the mother is homozygote for this mutation, the risk of NTD is 2-fold, if both the mother and fetus are homozygotes, the risk of NTD increased 6-7-fold. Heterozygotes have a slight increase in the risk of NTD.

Obviously folate/FA is a key factor in homocysteine metabolism, but vitamin B12, B2 and B6 have also role in this biological mechanism (Figure) and it may explain a higher efficacy of a multivitamin including these 4 "fetal protective" B vitamins as folic acid alone in the reduction of NDT. The use of multivitamins containing FA and other B vitamins in the Hungarian RCT and CCT and in the study of Smithells et al. showed a higher efficacy (about 90%) in the reduction of NTD than the MRC Vitamin Study using a high dose of FA alone (71%) and Chinese-US study using a low dose of FA (41-79%). The usual argument against the use of other vitamins is that the supplementation group of "other vitamins" in the MRC Vitamin Study did not result in a significant reduction in recurrent NTD. However, it is worth mentioning that there was a 40% reduction (2.6% vs. 4.3%) in the recurrent NTD near to the level of significance after the supplementation of other vitamins.

Animal experiments showed that the component CCA of fetal alcohol syndrome is preventable by folic acid (Serrano et al., 2010). However, the origin of isolated common CCA types such as ventricular septal defect is also explained by gene-environmental interaction. Several genes and environmental factors contribute to the origin of CCAs, one of them may be hyperhomocysteinemia. Kapusta et al (1999) found a higher plasma homocysteine level in mothers who delivered infants with CCA compared to the mothers of healthy babies. Later an association was reported of a higher plasma homocysteine level and MTHFR-gene polymorphism with CCA, though the recent evaluation of 13 eligible studies did not reveal association with the risk of CCAs with fetal (OR with 95% CI: 1.3, 0.97–1.73) and maternal (OR with 95% CI: 1.2, 0.83–1.74) MTHFR TT genotypes (van Beynum et al., 2007). However, functional polymorphism in folate-related genes increases the risk of having a fetus with CCA when maternal obesity or smoking habit is present (Hobbs et al., 2010).

Other Effects of Folic Acid/Multivitamins in Pregnant Women

The great majority of the women in the Hungarian RCT were healthy and not malnourished; therefore this RCT was appropriate to study several other effects of periconceptional FA-containing multivitamin supplementation.

During the preconceptional multivitamin supplementation the female cycle became more regular, i.e. the variance was lower (Dudás et al., 1995). Thus, multivitamin supplementation may have a beneficial effect for women with irregular menstrual cycles.

There was no difference in the sexual activity (measured by the rate of weekly sexual intercourse) of couples between the multivitamin and the no multivitamin groups in the preconceptional period (Czeizel et al., 1996a). However, only women were supplemented and sexual activity is often determined by males.

A 7% higher rate of conceptions occurred in women within one year who were treated with the multivitamin preconceptionally compared with those who were not supplemented. The time taken to become pregnant was slightly but significantly shorter in the multivitamin group (Czeizel et al., 1996b).

The rate of multiple births, namely twins was about 40% higher after periconceptional multivitamin supplementation (Czeizel et al., 1994). The higher rate of twin conceptions could not be explained by maternal factors (age, parity) or by a higher rate of infertility drug use (Czeizel et al., 1994a), and in vitro fertilization did not occur among these pregnant women (Czeizel et al., 1994b). This finding was confirmed later in the USA (Werler et al., 1997) and Sweden (Erickson et al., 2001), but not in China (Zhu et al., 2003). However, the incidence of twins is lowest in the Oriental race (including Chinese population) and Chinese people have an extremely high occurrence of TT genotype of MTHFR-gene (55%) (Botto and Yang, 2000), and this genotype associates with a very low dizygotic twin rate (Hasbergen et al., 2000). These conflicting data stimulated us to check the large material of the Hungarian Case-Control Surveillance of Congenital Abnormalities, including 38,151 controls without CA (Czeizel and Vargha, 2004). There was a somewhat higher prevalence of multiple pregnancies both after periconception high doses (mainly 6 mg) of FA and FA (0.1-1.0 mg) containing multivitamin supplementation. A systematic review of the recent literature, July 1994 to July 2006 resulted in the conclusion: "Overall…there is possible evidence for a relationship between periconceptional folic acid intake and increased twinning" (Muggli and Halliday, 2007).

A significantly lower rate of severe (treated) morning sickness, i.e. nausea and vomiting in early pregnancy occurred after periconception multivitamin supplementation (3.0% versus 6.6% in the no multivitamin group) (Czeizel et al., 1993).

There was no difference in gestational age at birth and birth weight, in addition the rate of preterm birth and low birthweight newborns of live-born babies of mothers with or without supplementation of the multivitamin in the periconception period (Czeizel et al., 1994c).

Postnatal somatic (body weight, body length, head circumference) and mental (measured by three tests) development until one (Czeizel and Dobó, 1994) and six years (Dobó and Czeizel, 1998) of age did not show any significant difference between the multivitamin and no multivitamin groups. However, it is necessary to stress that our pregnant women used a FA-containing multivitamin until the 12th gestational week, and main part of brain development is in the second, but mainly in the third trimester if pregnancy.

There was no difference in maternal weight gain between the multivitamin and no multivitamin groups before and during pregnancy (Czeizel, 1993a). In Hungary this possible side effect caused the major concern among females.

All other possible side effects were monitored continuously. The number of female participants in the Coordinating Center of the HPS was 14,540 until January, 1999 and patients with megaloblastic and pernicious anemia have not been recorded among these reproductive aged women. Of 14,540 female participants, four (0.03%) had severe allergic exanthema, and of these 4, three discontinued the use of multivitamin (all of them had a history of drug induced allergic diseases). Among all other possible side effects, constipation (1.8 vs. 0.8%) and diarrhoea (1.4 vs. 0.4%) were reported a somewhat more often after multivitamin supplementation in the preconception period (Czeizel, 1993a).

Practical Use of Folic Acid/Folate and Multivitamins during Pregnancy

Our hope is that the previous historical review can show that theoretically there was a breakthrough in the prevention of NTD, CCAs and likely some other CAs due to periconception FA/multivitamin supplementation. However, the beneficial effect of this important new preventive method has not been used appropriately in the medical practice.

There are four main possibilities to use FA/folate and appropriate multivitamins for women of childbearing age who are capable of becoming pregnant.

1. Consumption of Folate-Rich and other Vitamin-Rich Diet

The usual daily intake of folate is about 0.16-0.20 mg/d in Hungary (Czeizel and Susánszky, 1996) and this consumption is not significantly higher in other countries (Department of Health, UK, 2000). McPartlin et al. (1993) estimated that the optimal daily intake of folate/FA in the pre- and postconception period is about 0.66 mg per day for the prevention of NTD. Thus, the difference is about 0.50 mg and it is difficult to imagine about a 3.5 fold increase in folate intake every day in anticipation of conception, which means about 15 servings of broccoli on each day (Bower and Wald, 1995). Furthermore, some part of dietary folate is lost through cooking and processing. Finally, an extreme increase in the consumption of extra folate from natural food is relatively ineffective at increasing folate status (Cuskelly et al., 1996).

In conclusion, it is an important task to advise all women to have a folate- and other vitamin-rich diet from the preconception time onwards to prevent NTD and others CA, but it is necessary to stress that folate-rich diet alone cannot completely neutralize the genetic predisposition for these CAs.

2. Periconception Folic Acid and/or Multivitamin Supplementation

Good evidence is available to advise all women capable of becoming pregnant to have periconception (i.e., 2-3 month before and until 3 months after conception) FA or FA-containing multivitamin supplementation to reduce the occurrence of NTD and CCAs.

Thus periconception use of FA or multivitamins it would be a simple and useful approach, nevertheless this opportunity is missed frequently. The main cause is that 30-70% of pregnancies are unplanned, e.g. this figure is about 50% in the United States and Hungary. If women have unplanned pregnancies and are not using a supplement routinely, they cannot take advantage of this new preventive method during the preconception period. The explanation is clear, the beginning of first missed menstrual period overlaps with the 15th postconception day, i.e. when the possible pregnancy is recognized, the closing of neural-tube had started.

There are two public health tasks to help prospective pregnant women in order to increase their use of periconception FA or multivitamins. The first is a strong and widespread educational campaign to suggest the start of the use of

FA or multivitamins immediately after the discontinuation of oral contraceptive pills or other contraceptive methods when couples decide to have a baby. However, unfortunately these campaigns have had only a limited success in all countries (Busby et al., 2005; Botto et al., 2005; Neville and de Walle, 2010).

The second important task is to establish a network of pre-or *periconception care* within the primary heath care (Healthy People, USA, 2000). The Hungarian Periconception Service (HPS) was launched in 1984 (Czeizel et al., 1998) and the Hungarian RCT and CCT – presented previously - were based on the HPS. We prefer to use the term periconception instead of usual preconception because prenatal care usually begins in about the 7-12th week of pregnancy, but the most sensitive and vulnerable time of fetal development is from the 3rd postconception week until the 8th week, and this period is omitted from medical health service, thus embryos are uncared and, in general, unprotected. The preparation for conception is an appropriate period to stop smoking, alcohol drinking, narcotic and unnecessary drug uses with hazards to germ cells and later the fetus, in addition an optimal time for the launch of preconception FA or multivitamin supplementation.

Our Hungarian experiences have shown that periconception care is feasible and economical, in addition to providing an appropriate opportunity for nutritional interventions as well (Czeizel et al., 2005).

However, there are two debated questions. The first is connected with the choice of *FA alone or FA-containing multivitamins*. As the previously mentioned intervention trials showed, FA-containing multivitamins seem to be more effective in the prevention of NTD, though obviously the use of FA alone is more simple and cheaper. Another argument for the use of FA-containing multivitamins that this supplementation is effective for the reduction of CCAs and some other CAs, but there are very limited data concerning a similar preventive effect of FA alone for these CAs.

Another important question is the *optimal dose of folic acid*. The upper tolerable dose of folate-FA for healthy persons including pregnant women is 1 mg by the US Institute of M (1998) and the European Commission Scientific Committee on Food (2000). Thus it is necessary to differentiate the physiological dose of folic acid (less than 1 mg daily) for preventive purposes in healthy persons and the pharmacological dose of folic acid (more than 1 mg daily) for the treatment of patients. Experts in the USA based upon the Hungarian RCT and some observational studies recommended that "all women of childbearing age who are capable of becoming pregnant should consume 0.4 mg of folic acid per day for the purpose of reducing their risk of having a pregnancy affected with spina bifida or other NTD" (CDC, 1992) and this recommendation was subsequently followed by several countries, though there was no scientific evidence for this dose in 1992. McPartlin et al. (1993) suggested that the optimal daily intake of folate/FA in the pre- and postconception period is about 0.66 mg per day for the prevention of NTD. Thus, the recommended intake of folate/FA advised to a woman of childbearing age, who is sexually active, is daily 0.70 mg (Food Safety Authority of Ireland, 2006). In addition Daly et al (1993) demonstrated that the lowest risk of having a child with NTD was related to red blood cell folate concentration of 906 nmol/L or more. However, it was not reached within 4 weeks after the previously recommended 0.4 mg FA supplementation, practically 8-12 weeks are needed to reach the recommended level of 906 nmol/L while the use of 0.8 mg FA resulted in necessary red blood cell folate concentration at 4.2±3.5 weeks (Brämswig et al., 2009). Thus obviously the previously recommended and widely used 0.4 mg dose of FA is not correct.

Thus we recommend 1.0 mg of folate/FA daily for all pre- and pregnant women, by the consumption of 0.2-0.3 mg folate through diet, and by supplementation of 0.7-0.8 mg FA (U.S. Preventive Service Task Force, 2009; Czeizel and Bánhidy, 2011).

The optimal dose of folic acid for the *reduction of recurrent NTD risk* is the third question. There is an international consensus due to the results of the MRC Vitamin study (1991) that 4 mg of folic acid is the best for this preventive effort. However, the study of Smithells et al (1980, 1989) also clearly demonstrated the high efficacy (about 90%) reduction in the recurrent NTD by a multivitamin containing 0.36 of FA. The results of the MRC Vitamin showed about 70% reduction in recurrent NTD after the use of 4 mg FA. In the data set of the Hungarian CCT 34 informative offspring had previous sibs or parents with NTD without recurrence in the supplemented cohort by a multivitamin containing 0.8 mg FA (Czeizel et al., 2004).

3. Food Fortification

Food fortification seems to be the most practical means of supplementation with FA and other vitamins for women with unplanned pregnancies. This public health initiative is comparable to the prevention of goiter by the addition of iodine to salt.

In February 1996, the US Department of Health and Human Services (1996) ordered food fortification with FA of all cereal grain products at a level of 0.14 mg/100 g beginning January 1998. This adds only about 0.1 mg FA to the average daily diet of women of reproductive age, and there was a 26% reduction in the total (birth + fetal) prevalence of NTD (Honein et al., 2001; Williams et al., 2002). The estimated benefit-cost ratio of U.S. FA fortification is 40:1 (Grosse et al., 2005), thus the estimated economic benefit in U.S. dollars is 312-425 million annually. Canada also introduced a mandatory flour fortification with FA (0.15 mg/100 of white flour) in September 1998 and 42% reduction was found in the total prevalence of NTD (De Wals et al., 2002) and 6 % reduction in the birth prevalence of CCAs (Ionescu-Ittu et al., 2009). Later many others countries introduced the mandatory flour fortification, and as far as we know, at present this public health project is existing in 57 countries. However, mandatory flour or other food fortifications with FA are not available in European countries.

The mandatory flour fortification would be especially important for the large proportion of women with lower levels of education and income who, in general, have difficulties buying more expensive foods rich in folate and other vitamins and who have more frequently unplanned pregnancies.

Our major concern regarding this approach is the low dose of FA and the lack of vitamin B12. On the one hand there is well-known dose-effect relation in the preventive effect of FA for NTD, and it explains that some experts recommended the use of 5 mg FA (Wald et al., 2001, Koren and Goh, 2007). In our opinion 0.8 mg is a good compromise. On the other hand vitamin B12 is an independent risk factor in the origin of NTD (Kirke et al.,1993), and the combination of FA and vitamin B12 can prevent the so-called "masking effect" of folic acid in patients with pernicious anemia (Oakley, 1997).

However, there are two other opposite opinions regarding flour fortification with FA. Results of studies showed that folate deficiency is a precancerous state, but recent data suggested the possible carcinogenic effect of high doses of FA as well. Thus there may be U-shaped risk of cancer in connected with the doses of FA (Fenech, 2001). Therefore some experts did not recommend the introduction of flour fortification by FA because it may associate with risk in older people with precancerous lesions, e.g. in the colon (Osterhues at al., 2009). The opposite opinion is based on the good experiences of flour fortification in USA and Canada, thus Oakley (2002) declared that inertia on FA fortification is a public health malpractice.

4. Combination of Oral Contraceptives and Folate

Obviously periconception FA or FA-containing multivitamin supplementation requires planned conception and the proportion of females who are preparing their conception is between only 30% and 75% in different countries. Thus obviously we have to do our best to find alternative approaches and the combination of oral contraceptive pill with FA or folate seems to be another option (Holzgreve, 2010). Both natural folate and synthetic FA after their intakes are converted to 5-MTHF and this is the predominant folate form usually found in blood plasma. This nature-identical folate of 5-MTHF was synthesized as 6S-5-MTHF (methylfolate or levomefolate). Recently the US FDA (Food and Drud Administration) has approved a new medicinal product comprising of drospirenone and ethinyl-estradiol as contraceptive components and levomefolate calcium as folate component.

Five advantages can be expected from this new approach (Czeizel at al., 2011).

i. Overall 30-50% of women between the ages of 15 and 49 take the oral contraceptives in most Western European countries (Szarevski, 2010). Information on the beneficial effects of FA or FA-containing multivitamins could be provided on the contraceptives packet. Thus our hope is that the user of this medicinal product will have a better knowledge to understand that the start of the use of FA or multivitamins immediately after the discontinuation of oral contraceptive pills is necessary when couples decide to have a baby.
ii. A well-known fact that the compliance of pill use is not prefect, therefore inadvertent ‘accidental’ conception may occur about 2% of women who use contraceptive pills. Thus, the parallel use of folate is important for the prevention of NTD of their fetuses.
iii. Studies showed that 42% of women who discontinued pill use did not have consultation with their health care provider (Rosenberg and Waugh, 1998). In addition about 60% of young females who used oral contraceptives and stopped in order to have their first pregnancy, had no connection with gynecologists in Hungary (Czeizel et al., 1998)
iv. The European Active Surveillance Study (EURAS) evaluated 2000 women who stopped taking oral contraceptives in order to become pregnant (Cronin et al., 2009) and 31% were pregnant in the first

month after stopping oral contraceptive use and 46% after 3 months. In another study conception occurred within 2 months after the cessation of oral contraceptives use in 30-40% of all pregnancies and within 4 months in 50-60% (Dunson et al., 2004). Thus an important benefit is for women who discontinued the use of combination of contraceptive pills and folate that they have a higher blood folate level – though, of course, - with a decline parallel with the time. This "post-use effect" may be useful to reduce the risk of NTD. However, while the plasma folate level reflects the intake of folate/FA in previous days, red blood cell folate level shows a more constant, characteristic level because its change is slowly within the 120-day life of erythrocytes. Thus it is understandable that plasma folate concentration has a faster decrease after the discontinuation of oral contraceptives (Baker et al., 2009), and it is important to know that the cells of the fetus are exposed to circulating plasma folate.

v. 6S-5-MTHF and FA showed comparable physiological activity, bioavailability and absorption (Pietrzik et al., 2010). Thus as the equimolar dose of 6S-5-MTHF appears to be at least as effective as FA in increasing maternal red blood cell folate concentration in women of childbearing age (Lamers et al., 2006; Pietrzik et al., 2007). On the other hand human data of controlled epidemiological studies regarding the preventive effect of 6S-5-MTHF for NTD and other CAs are not available.

In conclusion the expected benefits of combined oral contraceptive with folate can be defined while it is difficult to estimate the possible unexpected risks. Neverthless, the introduction of this new medicinal product for the prevention of NTD in the most important target group, women of reproductive age, seems to be promising.

As we mentioned previously, the beneficial effect of this important new preventive method has not been used appropriately in the medical practice, though there are 4 options for the use FA/folate and appropriate multivitamins in women of childbearing age who are capable of becoming pregnant. Nevertheless, unfortunately, the elective termination of pregnancy after the prenatal diagnosis of NTD in fetuses is used much more frequently, than the truth prevention of these defects though the efficacy of these methods is similar, vitamin supplementation is much cheaper and is not associated with psychological problem and moral dilemma. Thus we have to do our best to accept and utilize the truth of the old English proverb: "An ounce of prevention is better than a pound of care"

Preterm Birth Preventive Effect of Folic Acid

In Hungary most pregnant women use high doses of folic acid during pregnancy mainly after the first visit in the prenatal care clinics (Czeizel and Vargha, 2004). However, the question is frequently raised whether it is worth continuing this supplement after the first trimester of pregnancy or not. Meta-analyses of supplementation studies recommended further researches to measure the effect of dietary folate or FA intake during pregnancy on reducing the rate of preterm delivery and low birthweight as an "urgent priority" (Mohammed 1993; Haider and Bhutta, 2006). On the other hand recently the fetal weight promoting effect of FA and/or multivitamins has been stated by some medical doctors as an argument against this preventive method, because the large birthweight may associate with a higher risk for birth complications of newborns.

The population-based dataset of the *Hungarian Case-Control Surveillance of Congenital Abnormalities (HCCSCA)* (Czeizel et al., 2001) was appropriate to test the hypothesis regarding the possible fetal growth promoting and/or preterm birth reduction effect of FA supplementation during pregnancy, particularly in the third trimester, i.e. during the FA. Controls (henceforth *newborns*) were selected from the National Birth Registry of the Central Statistical Office. In general two newborns were matched to every case with CA selected from the Hungarian Congenital Abnormality Registry according to sex, birth week, and district of parents' residence. Newborns from multiple pregnancies were excluded from this analysis.

Data of maternal variables and exposures were obtained from three sources: (i) an explanatory letter was mailed to mothers immediately after the selection of newborns asking them to send us the *prenatal maternity logbook* and other *medical records* regarding the study pregnancy and these medical documents were sent back within 3 weeks. Prenatal care was mandatory for pregnant women in Hungary (if somebody did not visit prenatal care clinic, she did not receive a maternity grant and leave), thus nearly 100% of pregnant women visited prenatal care clinics, on average 7 times, in their pregnancies. The first visit was between the 6th and 12th gestational week, and obstetricians recorded, among other information, vitamin supplements in the prenatal maternity logbook. (ii) A structured *questionnaire* with a list of medicinal products (drugs and pregnancy supplements) and diseases, plus a printed informed consent form were also mailed to the mothers. Mothers were asked to read these enclosed lists as a memory aid before they filled in the questionnaire and to send back it with the signed informed consent.

The mean ± S.D. time elapsed between the birth and the return of the "information package" (questionnaire, logbook, discharge summary, signed informed consent) in our prepaid envelope was 5.2 ± 2.9 months. Overall, the necessary information was available in 83.0% of newborns.

Only one type of 3 mg FA tablet was available in Hungary during the study period. Different multivitamins had low doses of FA therefore these medicinal products were excluded from this analysis. In addition pregnant women supplemented both FA and multivitamins were also excluded. The reference group included pregnant women without FA and multivitamin supplementation before conception (at least 3 months) and during the study pregnancy.

Gestation age was calculated from the first day of the last menstrual period, and was evaluated with birth weight on the basis of discharge summaries of inpatient obstetric clinics. The rate of low birthweight (< 2,500 g) and preterm births (< 37 weeks) were estimated on the gestation age at delivery and birth weight of newborns.

Among confounders, we evaluated maternal age, birth order (parity), maternal employment status which showed a correlation with education and income thus was used as indicator of socioeconomic status of pregnant women in the total data set.

There were 2,146,574 births in Hungary during the study period (19800-1996). Our sample included 38,151 newborns, thus represented 1.8% of Hungarian births, and 19,102 (50.0%) had mothers with FA supplementation. These pregnant women used 1-3 tablets of FA per day (1 tablet: 22%, 2 tablets: 69%, 3 tablets: 9%), thus the estimated daily dose was 5.6 mg. Of 19,102 pregnant women with FA supplement, 12,778 (66.9) had medically recorded FA use in the prenatal maternity logbook and 6,293 (92.9%) had their first pregnancy.

The mean maternal age was the same in the FA (23.2 ± 4.0 yr) and the reference groups (23.2 ± 4.2 yr) with nearly similar mean birth order (1.6 ± 0.8 vs. 1.7 ± 0.6). The proportion of high socioeconomic status was larger in the FA group (42.3%) than in the reference sample (38.0%). The proportion of smokers (15.8%) was lower in pregnant women with FA supplementation than in the reference group (19.1%) during the study pregnancy. The proportion of regular drinkers was about 1% in the study groups.

The occurrence of maternal acute (e.g. fever related influenza) and chronic (such as diabetes mellitus, epilepsy, etc) diseases, in addition the spectrum and occurrence of different drug treatments did not show significant difference between FA and reference groups.

The main objective of this analysis was to evaluate the pregnancy/birth outcomes of pregnant women with FA supplement and the reference group. Student t test and OR with 95% CI were used for statistical analyses, gestational age and preterm birth were adjusted for maternal age and socioeconomic status, in addition birth order, while it was completed with gestational age in birth weigh and low birthweight newborns.

The sex ratio of newborns did not show difference between FA and reference groups. The mean gestation age at delivery was 39.5 $\pm$ 2.0 and 39.2 $\pm$ 2.1 in pregnant women with FA supplementation and in the reference group, respectively. Thus mean gestation age was 0.3 week longer after FA supplements during pregnancy than in the reference sample ($p < 0.0001$). The mean birth weight was 3,294 $\pm$ 501 g in the newborns of pregnant women with FA supplements and 3,262 $\pm$ 509 in the reference group, i.e., it was only 32 grams larger in the group of FA alone (p=0.82). The rate of preterm births was 7.6% in the group of pregnant women with FA supplementation while 11.1% in the reference group, and this 3.5% difference was significant (OR with 95% CI: 0.68, 0.63-0.73). The rate of low birthweight was also lower in the FA group (5.1%) than in the reference group (6.8%) but this 1.1% difference was not significant (OR with 95% CI: 0.88, 0.62-1.14).

In the next step the possible association of longer gestation age and particularly the lower rate of preterm births after FA supplementation was analyzed according to different trimesters based on only prospectively and medically recorded supplementation (to exclude possible recall bias) and primiparae (to exclude pregnant women with possible previous preterm birth). The onset and end of supplementation were recorded in the prenatal maternity logbook or reported by mothers in the questionnaire according to gestation month.

Table 2 summarizes the data of medically recorded FA supplementation in primiparae. The longest gestation age and lowest rate of preterm birth was found after FA supplementation during the entire pregnancy, i.e. I-III trimesters (39.8 wk and 4.9%) and the II-III trimesters (39.9 wk and 3.8%), followed by the III trimester alone (39.5 wk and 7.6%). This trend resulted in 39.8 wk of mean gestation age and 4.8% rate of preterm birth in the group of

III trimester together (III + II-III + I-III trimesters). Our data suggest that the third trimester is a key time window of FA supplement use for the reduction of preterm births. In addition it is worth mentioning that mean gestation age was shorter and rate of preterm birth was higher if pregnant women were supplemented with FA only during the first trimester and particularly only during the second trimester. The mean birth weight increased by 13, 2 and 62 g after FA supplementation in the first, second and third trimester compared to the reference value, respectively.

Table 2. Pregnancy outcomes in primiparae with prospectively recorded use folic acid supplement alone by trimesters of use

Trimester of use	No.	Gestation age (wk)**		Birth weight (g)***		Preterm birth **		Low birth-weight ***	
		Mean	S.D.	Mean	S.D.	No.	%	No.	%
Reference*	7,319	39.2	2.1	3,216	486	864	11.8	416	5.7
I.	1,118	39.1	2.1	3,229	478	133	11.9	54	4.8
p/OR		0.50		0.19		1.00 (0.82-1.21)		0.81 (0.58-1.13)	
II.	896	38.8	2.3	3,218	505	136	15.2	49	5.5
p/OR		<0.001		0.49		1.31 (1.04-1.85)		0.96 (0.76-1.22)	
III.	514	39.5	1.8	3,278	481	39	7.6	26	5.1
p/OR		<0.001		0.14		0.62 (0.45-0.87)		0.89 (0.40-1.66)	
I-II.	88	39.4	2.1	3,241	480	9	10.2	7	8.0
p/OR		0.26		0.77		0.86 (0.43-1.72)		1.40 (0.31-4.11)	
II-III.	1,622	39.9	1.7	3,257	455	61	3.8	68	4.2
p/OR		<0.0001		0.004		0.29 (0.23-0.38)		0.74 (0.34-1.27)	
I-III.	2,055	39.8	1.8	3,270	494	101	4.9	115	5.6
p/OR		<0.0001		0.30		0.39 (0.32-0.49)		0.98 (0.51-1.58)	
Total	6,293	39.5	1.9	3,253	482	479	7.6	319	5.1
p/OR		<0.0001		0.86		0.62 (0.55-0.70)		0.89 (0.68-1.13)	
III. together	4,191	39.8	1.8	3,266	478	201	4.8	209	5.0
(I-III,II-III,III)		<0.0001		0.08		0.38 (0.33-0.45)		0.88 (0.56-1.27)	

* pregnant women without FA/MV supplementation.
** adjusted for maternal age, socioeconomic status.
*** adjusted for maternal age, socioeconomic status and gestation age.
Bold numbers show significant positive associations.

The maternal demographic and social data are not shown in Table 2, but it is worth mentioning that the largest proportion of high socioeconomic status was seen in pregnant women with I trimester, i.e. early FA supplementation which included preconception use of FA in pregnant women.

Thus our findings showed that fetal growth promoting effect of FA supplements was limited (37 g during entire pregnancy, and 62 g in the third trimester), thus does not seem to be important from clinical aspect. In addition this minor increase in the birth weight can be explained mainly by the longer gestation age. On the other hand we found an obvious preterm birth reducing effect of FA supplements particularly in the third trimester.

The Hungarian rate of preterm births is high among European countries (Bjerkedahl et al., 2004) though similar to the U.S. rate (Goldenberg et al., 2008). Mothers who delivered prematurely generally have lower dietary folate intake and/or FA supplement during pregnancy (Scholl et al., 1996), though folate demand is increased in pregnancy (McPartlin et al., 1993). Thus without adequate dietary intake of folate or FA supplementation, concentrations of folate in maternal plasma and red blood cells decrease from the 5th months of pregnancy onwards (Cikot et al., 2001).

Mothers who delivered prematurely had lower dietary folate intake (Siega-Riz et al., 2000) and higher blood homocysteine levels (Vollset et al., 2000). FA-containing multivitamin supplementation in the periconception period (Shaw et al., 1997) or during the first and second trimesters of pregnancy (Scholl et al., 1997) resulted in a reduction of preterm births. However, there was no lower rate of preterm birth and low birthweight newborns after the periconception FA-containing multivitamin supplementation in the Hungarian RCT (Czeizel et al., 1994c). A small reduction was found in the rate of preterm births and low birthweight newborns among California infants after compulsory food fortification with folic acid (Shaw et al., 2004). The association of short interpregnancy intervals with higher rate of preterm birth was also explained by the role of folate depletion during pregnancy and postpartum period (Smits and Essed, 2001). A recent US study showed in 34,480 women with low-risk singleton pregnancies that preconception FA supplementation for 1 year or longer associated with a 70% decrease in the risk of spontaneous preterm delivery between 20 and 28 gestation weeks and a 50% reduction in preterm deliveries of 28 to 32 weeks. After 32 weeks, no significant effect of preconception FA supplementation on preterm delivery was found (Bukowski and Malone, 2009).

The first hypothesis for the explanation of preterm reduction due to FA supplementation during the third trimester in our study was based on the well-known fact that pregnant women who used vitamin supplements may be associated with a better preconception and/or prenatal care and/or the better lifestyle. This hypothesis was supported by a somewhat lower socioeconomic status and somewhat higher rate of smokers in the group of unsupplemented pregnant women. However, we considered these confounders at the calculations of adjusted OR, thus cannot explain the trimester dependent trend after FA supplementation. Our present hypothesis is that the reduced maternal folate status may be associated with elevated homocysteine related placental vasculopathy (van den Molen et al., 2000; Ferguson et al., 2001; Eskes, 2002) which can be neutralized with high dose of FA supplementation during pregnancy particularly in the third trimester. Johnson et al (2005) showed an interaction between a pregnant woman's dietary folate intake and the presence or absence of a deletion allele in a folate-metabolizing gene explaining the different genetic predisposition due to folate deficiency during pregnancy.

In conclusion the high dose of FA supplementation during pregnancy particularly in the third trimester reduces the risk of preterm birth. Of 136 million total births per year worldwide, more than 4 million newborns die within the first days or weeks of life. The major causes of their death are preterm birth, birth asphyxia and infections (WHO, 2005). Thus, the reduction of preterm births by FA supplementation would be very important.

Conclusion

FA and FA-containing multivitamins using during the periconception period resulted in a breakthrough in the prevention of CAs, particularly NTD and CCAs, thus theoretically it is possible to reduce the occurrence of CAs by one-third. Unfortunately this good chance to help the wish of prospective parents to have healthy baby is not used widely in the medical practice though four possible approaches of this preventive method are available. In addition recent studies have shown that FA is able to reduce the rate of preterm birth as well. CAs and preterm births are the two major factors of infant mortality and handicaps; therefore we have to do our best to use FA and/or FA-containing multivitamins in the periconception period and later during pregnancy to protect the health of newborn infants.

References

Baker, DJ, de Jong-van den Berg, LTW, Fokkema, MR. (2009) Controlled study on folate status following folic acid supplementation and discontinuation in women of child-bearing age. *Ann. Clin. Biochem.* 46: 231-234.

Baker, H, Frank, O, Deangelis, B. et al (1981) Role of placenta in maternal-fetal vitamin transfer in humans. *Am. J. Obstet. Gynecol.* 141: 792-796.

Berry, RJ, Li, Z, Erickson, JD. et al (1999) Prevention of neural-tube defects with folic acid in China. China-US Collaborative Project for Neural Tube Defect Prevention. *N. Engl. J. Med.* 341: 1485-1490.

Bjerkedahl T, Czeizel AE, Hosmer DW. (1993) Birth weight of single livebirths and weight specific early neonatal mortality in Hungary and Norway. *Paediat. Perinat. Epidemiol.* 3: 129-140.

Bolander-Gouaille, C. (2002) Focus on Homocysteine and the Vitamins. Second edition, Springer, Paris.

Botto LD, Yang G. (2000) 5,10,methylenetetrahydrofolate reductase gene variants and congenital abnormalities. A HuGE review. *Am. J. Epidem.* 15: 862-877.

Botto LD, Khoury MJ, Mulinare J, Erickson JD (1996) Periconceptional multivitamin use and the occurrence of conotruncal heart defects. Results from a population-based case-control study. *Pediatrics* 98: 911-917.

Botto LD, Mulinare J, Erickson JD. (2000) Occurrence of congenital heart defects in relation to maternal multivitamin use. *Am. J. Epidemiol.* 151: 878-884.

Botto, LD, Lisi, A, Robert-Gnansia E. et al (2005) International retrospective cohort study of neural tube defects in relation to folic acid recommendation? Are the recommendation working? *Brit. Med. J.* 330: 571.

Bower, C, Wald, NJ. (1995) Vitamin B12 deficiency and the fortification of food with folic acid. *Eur. J. Clin. Nutr.* 49: 87-93.

Brämswig, S, Prinz-Langenohl, R, Lamers, Y. et al (2009) Supplementation with a multivitamin containing 800 microgram of folic acid shortens the time to reach the preventive red blood cell folate concentration in healthy women. *Int. J. Vitam. Nutr. Res.* 79: 61-70.

Bukowski, R, Malone. FD. (2009) Preconceptional folate supplementation and the risk of spontaneous preterm birth: a cohort study. *PLoS Med.* 2009; 6(5): e10000061

Busby, A, Abramsky, L, Dolk, H. et al (2005) Preventing neural tube defects in Europe: a missed opportunity. *Reprod. Toxicol.* 20: 393-402.

CDC (1992) Recommendations for the use of folic acid to reduce the number of cases of spina bifida and other neural tube defects. *MMWR* 41: 1233-1238.

Chanarin, I, Rothman, D, Ward, A, Perry, J. (1968) Folate status and requirement in pregnancy. *Brit. Med. J.* 2: 390-394.

Chanarin, I, MacGibbon, BM, O'Sullivan, WJ, Mollin, DL. (1959) Folic acid-deficiency in pregnancy: The pathogenesis of megaloblastic anaemia of pregnancy. *Lancet* 2: 634-639.

Cikot RJLM, Steegers-Theunissen RPM, Thomas CMG et al (2001) Longitudinal vitamin and homocysteine levels in normal pregnancy. *Br. J. Nutr.* 85: 49-58.

Cronin, M, Schellschmidt, I, Dinger, J. (2009) Rate of pregnancy after using drosperinone and other progestin-containing oral contraceptives. *Obstet. Gynecol.* 114: 616-622.

Cuskelly, GJ, McNulty, H, Scott, J.M. (1996) Effect of increasing dietary folate on red-cell folate: implications for prevention of neural tube defects. *Lancet* 347: 657-659.

Czeizel, AE (1993a). Randomized, controlled trial of the effect of periconceptional multivitamin supplementation on pregnancy outcome. In: Wharton BA (ed.): Maternal-Child Issues in Nutrition Wyeth-Ayerst Nutritional Seminar Series. Excerpta Medica, Princeton, NJ, 13-24.

Czeizel, AE (1993b). Prevention of congenital abnormalities by periconceptional multivitamin supplementation. *Brit. Med. J.* 306: 1645-1648.

Czeizel, AE (1996). Reduction of urinary tract and cardiovascular defects by periconceptional multivitamin supplementation. *Am. J. Med. Genet.* 62: 179-183.

Czeizel, AE (1998) Periconceptional folic acid-contanining multivitamin supplementation. *Eur. J. Obstet. Gynec. Reprod. Biol.* 75: 151-161.

Czeizel, AE (1999) Ten years of experience in the periconceptional care. *Eur. J. Obstet. Gynec. Reprod. Biol.* 89: 43-49.

Czeizel, AE. (2008) Specified critical period of different congenital abnormalities: A new approach for human teratology. *Congenit. Anom.* 48: 103-109.

Czeizel, AE. (2010) Definition, classification, prevalence and economic burden of neural tube defects. *Gynaec. Forum* 15: 9-12.

Czeizel, AE, Bánhidy, F. (2011) Vitamin supply in pregnancy for prevention of congenital abnormalities. *Current Opinion Clinical Nutr. Metab. Care* 14: 291-296.

Czeizel, AE, Dobó, M. (1994) Postnatal somatic and mental development after periconceptional multivitamin supplementation. *Arch. Dis. Child* 70: 229-233.

Czeizel, AE., Dudás, I. (1992) Prevention of the first occurrence of neural-tube defects by periconceptional vitamin supplementation. *N. Engl. J. Med.* 327: 1832-1835.

Czeizel, AE, Medveczki, E. (2003) Periconceptional multivitamin supplementation and multimalformed offspring. *Obstet. Gynecol.* 102: 1255-1261.

Czeizel, AE., Révész, C. (1970) Major malformation of the central nervous system in Hungary. *Br. J. Prev. Soc. Med.* 24: 205-222.

Czeizel, AE, Susánszky, E. (1994) Diet intake and vitamin supplement use of Hungarian women during the preconceptional period. *Int. J. Vitam. Nutr. Res.* 64: 300-305.

Czeizel, AE, Vargha, P. (2004) Periconceptional folic acid/multivitamin supplementation and twin pregnancy. *Am. J. Obstet. Gynecol.* 1891: 790-794.

Czeizel, AE, Dudás, I, Fritz, G et al. (1992) The effect of periconceptional multivitamin-mineral supplementation on vertigo, nausea and vomiting in the first trimester of pregnancy. *Arch. Gynecol. Obstet.* 251: 181-185.

Czeizel AE, Métneki J, Dudás I. (1994a) Higher rate of multiple births after periconceptional multivitamin supplementation. *N. Engl. J. Med.* 330: 1687-1688.

Czeizel AE, Métneki J, Dudás I. (1994b) The higher rate of multiple births after periconceptional multivitamin supplementation: An analysis of causes. *Acta Genet. Gemmellol.* 43: 175-184.

Czeizel AE, Dudás I, Métneki J. (1994c) Pregnancy outcomes in a randomized controlled trial of periconceptional multivitamin supplementation. Final report. *Arch. Gynecol. Obstet.* 255: 131-139.

Czeizel AE, Rockenbauer M, Susánszky E. (1996a) No change in sexual activity during periconceptional multivitamin supplementation. *Brit. J. Obst. Gynecol.* 1996; 103: 569-573.

Czeizel, AE, Métneki, J, Dudás I. (1996b) The effect of preconceptional multivitamin supplementation on fertility. *Int. J. Vitam. Nutr. Res.* 1996; 66: 55-58.

Czeizel AE, Tóth M, Rockenbauer M (1996c) A case-control analysis of folic acid supplementation during pregnancy. *Teratology* 53: 345-351.

Czeizel, AE, Dobó, M, Dudás, I. et al (1998) The Hungarian Periconceptional Service as a model for community genetics. *Community Genetics* 1: 252-259.

Czeizel AE, Tímár L, Sárközi A. (1999) Dose-dependent effect of folic acid on the prevention of orofacial clefts. *Pediatrics* 104: e66.

Czeizel AE, Rockenbauer M, Siffel Cs, Varga E. (2001) Description and mission evaluation of the Hungarian Case-Control Surveillance of Congenital Abnormalities, 1980-1996. *Teratology* 63: 176-185.

Czeizel, AE, Dobó, M, Vargha, P. (2004) Hungarian two-cohort controlled study of periconceptional multivitamin supplementation to prevent certain congenital abnormalities. *Birth Defects Res. Part A*. 70: 853-861.

Czeizel, AE, Gasztonyi, Z, Kuliev, A. (2005) Periconceptional clinics: A medical healthcare infrastructure of new genetics. *Fetal. Diagn Ther.* 20: 518-545.

Czeizel, AE, Puho, HE, Bánhidy, F. (2006) No association between periconceptional multivitamin supplementation and risk of multiple congenital abnormalities. A population-based case-control study. *Am. J. Med. Genet.* 140A: 2469-2477.

Czeizel, AE, Puho, HE, Langmar, Z et al (2010) Possible association of folic acid supplementation during pregnancy with reduction of preterm birth: a population-based study. *Eur. J. Obstet. Gynecol. Reprod. Biol.* 148: 135-140.

Czeizel, AE, Bártfai, Z, Bánhidy, F. (2011) Combined oral contraceptives with folate: What are the benefits? *Therapeutic Advances in Drug Safety* (in press).

Daily, L E, Kirke, P N, Molloy, A. et al (1993) Folate levels and neural tube defects. Implications for prevention. *J. Am. Med. Ass.* 274: 1698-1702.

Department of Health, UK (2000) Committee on Medical Aspects of Food and Nutrition Policy (COMA): Folic Acid and the Prevention of Disease, London.

De Wals, P, Tairou, F, Van Allen, M. et al (2007) Reduction in neural-tube defects after folic acid fortification in Canada. *N. Engl. J. Med.* 357: 135-142.

Dobó M, Czeizel AE. (1998) Longterm somatic and mental development of children after periconceptional multivitamin supplementation. *Eur. J. Pediat.* 157: 719-723.

Dudás, I, Rockenbauer, M, Czeizel AE. (1995) The effect of preconceptional multivitamin supplementation on the menstrual cycle. *Arch. Gynecol. Obstet.* 256: 115-123.

Dunson, DB, Baird, DD, Colombo, B. (2004) Increased infertility with age in men and women. *Obstet. Gynecol.* 103: 51-56.

Ek, J, Magnus, EM. (1981) Plasma and red blood cell folate during normal pregnancy. *Acta Obstet. Gynecol. Scand.* 60: 247-251.

Elwood, J M, Little, J, Elwood JH. (1992) Epidemiology and Control of Neural Tube Defects. Oxford University Press, Oxford.

Erickson A, Källen B, Aberg A. (2001) Use of multivitamins and folic acid in early pregnancy and multiple births in Sweden. *Twin. Res.* 4: 63-66.

Eskes TKAB (2002) Vascular disease in women. Folate and homocysteine. In:7 Massaro EJ, Rogers JM: Folate and Human Development. Humana Press. Totowa, NJ, pp. 299-328.

European Commission Scientific Committee on Food (2000) Tolerable upper limit levels for vitamins and minerals, Brussels.

Fenech, M. (2001) The role of folic acid and vitamin B12 in genomic stability of human cells. *Mutat. Res.* 475: 57-67.

Ferguson SE, Smith GN, Walker MC. (2001) Maternal plasma homocysteine levels in women with preterm premature rupture of membranes. *Med. Hypotheses* 56: 85-90.

Food Safety Authority of Ireland (2006) Report of the Committee on Folic Acid Food Fortification, Dublin.

Frosst, P, Blom, HJ, Milos, R. (1995) A candidate genetic risk-factor for vascular disease: a common mutation in methylenetetrahydrofolate reductase. *Nature Genet.* 10, 111-113.

Goh YI, Bollano E, Einarson, TR, Koren G. (2006) Prenatal multivitamin supplementation and rates of congenital anomalies: a meta-analysis. *J. Obstet. Gynaecol. Can.* 28: 680-689.

Goldenberg RL, Culhane JF, Iams JD, Romero R. (2008) Epidemiology of preterm birth. *Lancet* 371: 75-84.

Goyette, D, Summer, JS, Milos, R. (1994) Human methylenetetrahydrofolate reductase: isolation of cDNA, mapping and mutation identification. *Nature Genet.* 7: 195-200.

Grosse, SD, Waltzman, NJ, Romano, PS, Mulinare, J. (2005) Reevaluating the benefits of folic acid fortification in the United States: economic analysis, regulation, and public health. *Am. J. Publ. Health* 95: 1917-1922.

Haider BA, Bhutta ZA. (2006) Multiple-micronutrients supplementation for women during pregnancy. *Cochrane Database Syst. Rev.,* Oct 2006. 18 (4):CD004905.

Hasbargen U, Lohse P. Thaler CJ. (2000) The number of dichorionic twin pregnancies is reduced by the common MTHFR G77C→T mutation. *Hum. Reprod.* 15: 2059-2662.

Healthy People 2000 (2000) National health population and disease prevention objectives. US Department of Health and Human Service. *Public Health Service.* DHHS Publ. No. 91-502. 13.

Hibbard, BM. (1964) The role of folic acid in pregnancy with particular reference to anaemia, abruption and abortion. *J. Obstet. Gynecol.* 71: 529-542.

Hibbard, ED, Smithells, RW. (1965) Folic acid metabolism and human embryopathy. *Lancet* 1: 1254.

Hobbs CA, Cleves MA, Karim MA. (2010) Maternal folate-related gene environment interactions and congenital heart defects. *Obstet. Gynecol.* 116: 316-322.

Hoffbrand, AV. (2001) The history of folic acid. *Br. J. Haematol.* 113: 579-589.

Holzgreve, W. (2010) Adding folate to the pill to prevent neural tube defects. Gynaec Forum 15: 4-8.

Honein, MA, Paulozzi, LJ, Mathews, TJ. et al (2001) Impact of folic acid fortification of the US Food Supply on the occurrence of neural tube defects. *J. Am. Med. Ass.* 285: 2981-2986.

Ionescu-Ittu, R, Marelli, AJ, Mackie, AS, Pilote L. (2009) Prevalence of severe congenital heart disease after folic acid fortification of grain products. Time trend analysis in Quebec, Canada. *Brit. Med. J.* 338: 1673.

Johnson WG, Scholl TO, Spychala JR et al (2005) Common dihydrofolate reductase 19-base deletion allele: a novel risk factor for preterm delivery. *Am. J. Clin. Nutr.*. 81: 664-668.

Kapusta L, Haagmans MLM, Steegers EAP et al. (1999) Congenital heart defects and derangement of homocysteine metabolism. *J. Pediat.* 135: 773-774.

Kirke, PN, Molloy, AM, Daly, LE. et al (1993) Maternal plasma folate and vitamin B12 are independent risk factors for neural tube defects. *Q. J. Med.* 86: 703-708.

Koren, G, Goh, IY. (2007) Increasing folate supplementation for selected groups of Canadian women. *J. Obstet. Gynaecol. Can.* 29: 992-996.

Lamers, Y, Prinz-Langenohl, R, Brämswig, S, Pietrzik, K. (2006) Red blood cell folate concentrations increase more after supplementation with [6S]-methyltetrahydrofolate than with folic acid in women of childbearing age. *Am. J. Clin. Nutr.* 84: 156-161.

Landon, MJ, Eyre, DH, Hytten, FE. (1975) Transfer of folate to the fetus. *Br. J. Obstet. Gynecol.* 82 : 12-19.

Li D-K, Daling, JR, Mueller BA, et al. (1995) Periconceptional multivitamin use in relation to the risk of congenital urinary tract anomalies. *Epidemiology* 6: 212-218.

McPartlin, J, Halligan, A, Scott, JM. et al (1993) Accelerated folate breakdown in pregnancy. *Lancet* 341: 148-149.

Mészáros, M, Nagy, A, Czeizel AE (1975) Incidence of congenital heart diseases in Hungary. *Hum. Hered.* 25: 513-519.

Mohammed K. (1993) Routine folate supplementation in pregnancy. In: Enkin MW, Keirse MJCN, Renfreq MJ, Nielson JP (eds.) Pregnancy and Childbirth Module. *Cochrane Database Syst. Rev. Review*, No. 03158.

MRC Vitamin Study Research Group (1991) Prevention of neural tube defects: results of the Medical Research Council Vitamin Study. *Lancet* 338: 131-137.

Muggli, EE, Halliday, JH. (2007) Folic acid and risk of twinning: a systematic review of the recent literature, July 1994 to July 2006. *MJA* 186: 243-248.

Neville, AJ, de Walle, H E K. (2010) Prevention of neural tube defects by periconceptional folic acid supplementation in Europe. *Gynaec. Forum* 15: 16-20.

Nevin, NC, Seller, MJ. (1990) Prevention of neural tube defect recurrences. *Lancet* 1: 178-179.

Oakley, GP. (1997) Let's increased folic acid fortification and include vitamin B-12. *Am. J. Clin. Nutr.* 6: 1989-1990.

Oakley, GP. (2002) Inertia on folic acid fortification: Public health malpractice. *Teratology* 66: 44-54.

Osterhues, A, Holzgreve, W, Michels, KB. (2009) Shall we put the world on folate? *Lancet* 374: 959-960.

Pietrzik, K, Lamers, Y, Brämswig, S, Prinz-Langenohl, R. (2007) Calculation of red blood cell folate steady state conditions and elimination kinetics after daily supplementation with various folate forms and doses in women in childbearing age. *Am. J. Clin. Nutr.* 86: 1414-1419.

Pietrzik, K, Bailey, L, Shane, B. (2010) Folic acid and L-5-methyltetrahydrofolate: comparison of clinical pharmacokinetics and pharmacodynamics. *Clin. Pharmacokinet.* 49: 535-548.

Rosenberg, MJ, Waugh, M S. (1998) Oral contraceptives discontinuation: a prospective evaluation of frequency and reasons. *Am. J. Obstet. Gynecol.* 179: 577-582.

Scholl TO, Hediger ML, Schall JI et al (1996) Dietary and serum folate: their influence on the outcome of pregnancy. *Am. J. Clin. Nutr.* 63: 520-525.

Scholl TO, Hediger ML, Bendich A et al. (1997) Use of multivitamin/mineral prenatal supplements: influence on the outcome of pregnancy. *Am. J. Epidemiol.* 146: 134-141.

Serrano M, Han M, Brinez P, Linask KK (2010) Fetal alcohol syndrome: cardiac birth defects in mice and prevention with folate. *Am. J. Obstet. Gynecol.* 203:75.e75-75.e15.

Shaw GM, Liberman RF, Todoroff K, Wasserman CR. (1997) Low birth weight, preterm delivery, and periconceptional vitamin use. *J. Pediatr.* 130: 1013-1014.

Shaw GM, Carmincheael SL, Nelson V et al. (2004) Occurrence of low birthweight and preterm delivery among California infants before and after compulsory food fortification with folic acid. *Publ. Health Rep.* 119: 170-173.

Siega-Riz AM, Savitz SA, Zeisel SH et al (2000) Second trimester folate status and preterm birth. *Am. J. Obstet. Gynecol.* 191: 851-857.

Smithells, RW, Sheppard, S, Schorah, CJ. (1976) Vitamin deficiencies and neural tube defects. *Arch. Dis. Child* 51: 944-949.

Smithells, RW, Sheppard, S, Schorah, CJ. Et al. (1980) Possible prevention of neural tube defects by periconceptional vitamin supplementation. *Lancet* 1: 339-340.

Smithells, R W, Sheppard, S, Wild, J, Schorah, C J. (1989) Prevention of neural tube defect recurrences in Yorkshire: final report. *Lancet* 2: 498-499.

Smits LJM, Essed GGM. (2001) Short pregnancy intervals and unfavorable pregnancy outcomes: Role of folate depletion. *Lancet* 358: 2074-2077.

Szarevsky, A. (2010) Oral contraceptive and pregnancy planning. *Gynaec. Forum* 15: 23-28.

Tarusco D (ed.) (2004) Folic Acid: From Research to Public Health Practice. Rapporti ISTISAN 04/26, Roma.

Tolarova M. (1982) Periconceptional supplementation with vitamins and folic acid to prevent recurrence of cleft lip. *Lancet* 2: 217.

US Department of Health and Human Services. (1996) Food standards: amendment of standards of identity for enriched grain products to require addition of folic acid. *Federal Register* 61: 8781-8787.

US Institute of Medicine (1998): Dietary Reference Intakes: A Risk Assessment Model for Establishing Upper Intake Levels for nutrients. National Academy Press. Washington DC.

U.S. Preventive Service Task Force. (2009) Folic acid for the prevention of neural tube defects: U.S. Preventive Services Task Force recommendation statement. *Ann. Inter. Med.* 150: 626-631.

van Beynum IM, den Heijer M, Blom HJ, Kapusta L. (2007) The MTHFR 677C-T polymorphism and the risk of congenital heart defects: a literature review and meta-analysis. *QMJ* 100: 743-753.

van Beynum IM, Kapusta L, Bakker MK. (2010) Protective effect of periconceptional folic acid supplements on the risk of congenital heart defects: a registry-based case-control study in the northern Netherlands. *Eur. Heart J.* 31: 464-471.

van der Molen EF, Verbruggen B, Nokalova I. et al (2000) Hyperhomocysteinemia and other thrombotic risk factors in women with placental vasculopathy. *Br. J. Obstet. Gynaecol.* 2000; 107: 785-791.

Vollset SE, Refsum H, Irgens LM et al (2000) Plasma total homocysteine, pregnancy complications, and adverse pregnancy outcomes: The Hordaland Homocysteine Study. *Am. J. Clin. Nutr.* 71: 962-968.

Wald, NJ, Law, MR, Morris, JK, Wald, DS. (2001) Quantifying the effects of folic acid. *Lancet* 358: 2069-2073.

Werler, MM, Cragan, JD, Wasserman CR, et al (1997) Multivitamin supplementation and multiple births. *Am. J. Med. Genet.* 71: 93-96.

Werler MM, Hayes C, Louik C. (1999) Multivitamin use and risk of birth defects. *Am. J. Epidemiol.* 150: 675-682.

WHO Reg. 1 (2005) Make every mother and child count. http://www.who.int/whr/2005/download/en.

Wilcken, B, Bamforth, F, Li, Z. et al (2003) Geographical and ethnic variation of the 677C/T allele of 5,10 methylenetetrahydrofolate reductase (MTHFR): findings from over 7000 newborns from 16 areas world wide. *J. Med. Genet.* 40: 619-625.

Williams, LJ, Mai, C, Edmonds, LD. et al (2002) Prevalence of spina bifida and anencephaly during the transition to mandatoryfolic acid fortification in the United States. *Teratology* 66: 33-39.

Wills, L. (1931) Treatment of "pernicious anaemia" of pregnancy and "tropical anaemia" with special reference to yeast extract as a curative agent. *Brit. Med. J.* 1:1059-1064.

Wright, AJA, King, MJ, Finglas, PM. (2010) Folate-supplemented oral contraceptives: does 6S-5-methytetrahydrofolic acid (Metafolin[R]) offer advantages over folic acid? *Gynaec. Forum* 15: 29-32.

Yang Q, Khoury MJ, Olney RS, et al (1997) Does periconceptional multivitamin use reduce the risk for limb deficiency in offspring? *Epidemiology* 8: 157-161.

Zhu, L, Gindler, J, Wang, H. et al (2003) Folic acid supplementation during early pregnancy and likelihood of multiple births: a population-based cohort study. *Lancet* 361: 380-384.

In: Folic Acid
Editors: Mária Szabó and Eve Varga ISBN: 978-1-62100-867-5

Chapter II

The Role of Folic Acid in Psychiatric Disorders

***Josiane Budni*[1], *Patricia S. Brocardo*[2] and *Ana Lúcia S. Rodrigues*[1]**

[1]Departamento de Bioquímica, Centro de Ciências Biológicas, Universidade Federal de Santa Catarina, Florianópolis-SC, Campus Universitário, Trindade, Florianópolis-SC, Brazil
[2]Division of Medical Sciences, Island Medical Program, University of Victoria, Victoria, BC, Canada

Abstract

Folic acid is one of 13 essential vitamins that can be obtained from dietary sources or supplements. Despite a relative abundance of folic acid in food, its deficiency is frequent and can arise as a consequence of poor diet, chronic illness, drugs, malabsorption, and an increased demand. Noteworthy, folic acid is essential for the functioning of the nervous system, since it plays an important role in neuroplasticity and in the maintenance of neuronal integrity. Several studies have indicated that folic acid plays a role in the pathophysiology and/or treatment of neuropsychiatric disorders such as depression, bipolar disorder, and schizophrenia. Individuals with low blood levels of folic acid seem more prone to the development of these neuropsychiatric disorders. Moreover, this vitamin deficiency has been correlated with a reduced effectiveness or a poor response to medication such as antidepressants. Although several preclinical and clinical studies have indicated a link between folic acid deficiency and neuropsychiatric disorders, the mechanisms underlying the beneficial effects of folic acid against these diseases have not been fully elucidated. This chapter presents an overview of the preclinical and clinical studies that have pointed to the link between folic acid and psychiatric disorders highlighting the evidence for the use of folic acid supplementation as a potential therapeutic strategy for the treatment of these diseases.

Abbreviations

CSF	cerebrospinal fluid
cGMP	cyclic guonosine monophosphate
DHF	dihydrofolate
FST	forced swimming test
GSK-3β	glycogen synthase kinase-3
HRS	Hamilton Depression Rating Scale
5-HT1A receptor	5-hydroxytryptamine 1A receptor
5-HT2A/2C receptors	5-hydroxytryptamine 2A/2C receptors
MTHF	5-methyl-THF
MTHFR	methylenetetrahydrofolate reductase
NMDA	N-Methyl-D-aspartic acid
NO	nitric oxide
PPARγ	peroxisome proliferator-activated receptor-γ
RBC	red blood cell
THF	tetrahydrofolate
TST	tail suspension test
TNF-α	tumor necrosis factor alpha

Introduction

Depression, bipolar disorder and schizophrenia are neuropsychiatric conditions that contribute the most disability-adjusted life-years. It is estimated that around 14% of the global burden of disease has been attributed to these neuropsychiatric disorders. The incidence of these psychiatric disorders is estimated to be about 16% for major depression, 1% for bipolar disorder, and 2.6% for schizophrenia (Kessler et al., 2005; Prince et al., 2007). Therefore, it is of paramount importance to develop and test new therapeutic agents for the treatment of these disorders.

Folic acid is involved in the metabolism and functioning of many substances that are essential to nervous system function. These include purines and pyrimidines, DNA, RNA, aminoacids, phosphorous compounds, vitamin B12, methionine, S-adenosyl-methionine, dopamine, epinephrine, norepinephrine, and serotonin (Matson and Shea, 2003; Coppen and Bolander-Gouaille, 2005; Kronenberg et al., 2009; Lucock, 2011). Abnormalities in the metabolism of folic acid may affect nervous system functioning by altering the metabolism of these compounds. This notion is supported by the high incidence of folic acid deficiency associated with multiple psychiatric conditions, including depression, bipolar disorder and schizophrenia (Coppen and Bolander-Gouaille, 2005; Stahl, 2007; Miller, 2008; Krebs et al., 2009).

In this chapter, we provide an overview of the literature supporting a relationship between folic acid and depression, bipolar disorder and schizophrenia. We then discuss the potential implications of these findings for the prevention and treatment of these neuropsychiatric disorders.

Folic Acid and Depression

Depression is one of the most common psychiatric conditions seen in the general medical setting, affecting millions of individuals in the world. The efficacy of the current pharmacotherapy has not improved since the 1950s, with only 30–40% of the patients reaching complete remission of symptoms. Since complete remission followed by sustained recovery is the best therapeutic strategy (Lee et al., 2010), new therapeutic agents are currently been studied for the treatment of depression, including folic acid.

Folic acid (folate) plays an important role for the functioning of the nervous system (Coppen and Bolander-Gouaille, 2005; Reynolds, 2006; Stahl, 2007). The metabolism of folic acid in the cell is initiated by dihydrofolate reductase in a two-step reaction; in the first step, folic acid is converted into dihydrofolate (DHF); whereas in the second step dihydrofolate is further reduced to tetrahydrofolate (THF). THF can then be converted into additional physiological folates including 5-methyl-THF (MTHF), the form that is normally found in the circulation and in tissues. MTHF is also replenished by the conversion of folinic acid (5-formyltetrahydrofolate), an active metabolite of folic acid. Because de novo folic acid synthesis does not occur in the central nervous system, the maintenance of appropriate levels of folic acid and its metabolites in the brain depends on the adequate transport of this vitamin across the blood-brain barrier (Ramaekers and Blau, 2004). MTHF acts as a critical co-factor for the synthesis of the three monoamines (dopamine, norepinephrine, and serotonin) (Stahl, 2007). Moreover, folic acid is required to re-methylate homocysteine to methionine. Homocysteine is a non-protein-forming sulfur amino acid that in high concentrations can be neurotoxic (Lipton et al., 1997; Kruman et al., 2000).

A large body of clinical evidence has supported a link between folic acid deficiency and depression (Lazarou and Kapsou, 2010; Nahas and Sheikh, 2011). The main findings from these studies are summarized in Table 1and discussed below.

The relationship between folic acid and depression was first described in a study from Herbert et al. (1962) that found mental changes in a previously healthy man who was placed on a folic acid deficient diet. In support of this hypothesis, several studies have indicated that individuals showing psychiatric symptoms, such as depression and impaired cognitive functioning, also present low levels of folic acid in the plasma, serum, red blood cells (RBC), or cerebrospinal fluid (CSF) (Carney, 1967; Reynolds et al., 1970; Carney and Sheffield, 1978; Ghadirian et al., 1980; Abou-Saleh and Coppen, 1989; Bottiglieri et al., 2000; Lindeman et al., 2000). Importantly, patients with folic acid deficiency show a more severe psychiatric symptomatology than those reported in individuals with normal levels of this vitamin (Abou-Saleh and Coppen, 1989). Consistent with this notion, a study by Levitt and Joffe (1989) found that the duration of depressive episode was significantly correlated with low folic acid levels. Also, Bottiglieri et al. (2000) showed that around one third of severely depressed patients presented folic acid levels in RBC that are below the normal value (<150 μg/l). A different study indicated that patients with low dietary folic acid intake had a 67% increase in the risk of developing severe depressive symptoms when compared to patients with high dietary folic acid intake. Furthermore, this study also showed that in a Finish population of depressive male patients a lower consumption of folic acid was associated with the severity of their symptoms (Tolmunen et al., 2003). A recent study performed in Japanese adults (113 men and 79 women) with depressive symptoms, showed that low levels of folic acid in the serum were associated with an increased prevalence of depressive symptoms in men (Nanri et al., 2010). In contrast, some studies have reported no significant alterations in the Hamilton Depression Rating Scale (HRS) scores upon folic acid treatment (Williams et al., 2005; Ford et al., 2008; Walker et al., 2010). Moreover, a community-based population study found that only B6 and B12 vitamins, but not folic acid, can be predictive of depressive symptoms among older adults (Skarupski et al., 2010). Therefore, further studies are warranted in order to further evaluate the role of folic acid in depression.

It is noteworthy that folic acid deficiency leads to the accumulation of homocysteine. High levels of homocysteine in the central nervous system are associated with depression, dementia, Parkinson's disease, stroke, as well as negative symptoms of schizophrenia (Khanna, 2011). Moreover, it has been shown that folic acid deficiency can result in low levels of monoamines (serotonin, norepinephrine and dopamine) (Morris et al., 2008; Farah, 2009), which could contribute to the development of depressive symptoms (Krishnan and Nestler, 2010). It is also important to mention that genetic factors can also affect folic acid levels. One example is the inborn error in methionine synthase (an enzyme that converts folic acid to L-methylfolate) caused by a C677T-polymorphism (Arinami et al., 1997; Kelly et al., 2004; Lewis et al., 2006; Fathy et al., 2011).

Moreover, various studies indicate that deficiency of folic acid is linked to severe and longer lasting depressive relapses. A study conducted among 71 depressive patients with low serum folate status indicated an association between folic acid deficiency and depressive relapse during treatment with fluoxetine, indicating that depressive patients with low serum levels of folic acid can be at a higher risk of depressive relapse during the treatment of this disorder (Papakostas et al., 2004b). In agreement with this study, Astorg et al. (2008) showed that a low folic acid intake was associated with an increased risk of recurrent depression in middle-aged men. By contrast, it has been speculated whether this relationship between low levels of folic acid and depression is merely causal. A cross-sectional study found no correlation between low blood levels of folic acid and incidence of depressive symptoms, suggesting that low blood folic acid content may be a consequence rather than a cause of depressive symptoms (Kendrick et al., 2008).

Several studies have investigated the potential beneficial effects of folic acid supplementation in depressive patients. An early study from Botez et al. (1982) indicated that folic acid supplementation was beneficial in a neuropsychiatric syndrome characterized by mental changes, polyneuropathy, and depression. Folic acid supplementation (10 mg daily for a period of 7-11 months) significantly improved neurological symptoms of depression (Botez et al., 1984). Moreover, a study conducted by Godfrey et al. (1990) in depressive patients showed that supplementation of the current antidepressant therapy with methylfolate (bioactive form of folic acid; 15 mg daily for a period of 6 months) was associated with, enhanced clinical and social recovery of these subjects. Additionally, a study by Alpert et al. (2002) showed that an active form of folic acid, folinic acid (15 to 30 mg/day for eight weeks), enhanced the effects of selective serotonin reuptake inhibitors in refractory depressed patients.

Importantly, deficiency of folic acid is associated with a poorer response to classical antidepressants, such as fluoxetine, in depressive patients (Coppen and Bailey, 2000; Papakostas et al., 2004a; 2005). A study showed that hypofolatemia (i.e., low levels of folic acid) predisposes subjects to melancholic depression and poor response to fluoxetine (Fava et al., 1997). Moreover, the combined administration of 5'-methyltetrahydrofolic acid (50 mg) and a standard antidepressant (trazodone, 50 mg), twice daily significantly improved the clinical response of depressed patients with borderline or deficiency of folic acid. Indeed, in normofolatemic subjects the HRS scores were reduced following 3 weeks of treatment (Passeri et al., 1993). Further indicating that folic acid levels may be associated with the response to antidepressants, a study by Wesson et al. (1994) found that along with a significant correlation between red cell folic acid levels and severity of illness, there were significantly more responders (to a 5-week trial of desmethylimipramine) than non-responders who had an increase in RBC folic acid levels. In addition, a randomized, placebo controlled trial showed that folic acid (500μg daily, 10 week) plus fluoxetine (20 mg), improved the HRS scores, especially in women (Coppen and Bailey, 2000). Other similar study also found that folic acid can be an additional treatment for depressive hypofolatemic patients resistant to therapy with fluoxetine (Papakostas et al., 2004a). However, these patients show a delayed response to folic acid treatment when compared to eufolatemic subjects (Papakostas et al., 2005). A randomized study in twenty-seven patients that received fluoxetine (20 mg) and folic acid (10 mg/day) or fluoxetine and placebo alone for a period of 6 weeks, was also performed. The HRS scores were reduced in these patients. Furthermore, considering that folic acid is an important component of the endogenous defense system and it may elevate antidepressant responses, Resler et al. (2008) investigated the participation of lymphocyte serotonergic system in folic acid-supplemented depressed patients. The authors observed that treatment with a combination of folic acid plus fluoxetine reduced the homocysteine status and induced accumulation of serotonin in the lymphocytes, probably modifying the functioning of these cells in depression. Nevertheless, a community-based study that involved older adults with depressive symptoms provided no clear evidence for the potentiation of the effects of antidepressant medication by combining it with folic acid plus vitamin B12 (Christensen et al., 2011).

It is also important to consider that dietary supplementation or consumption of these B-vitamins (folic acid, B-6 and B-12) has been reported to prevent depression after stroke. In a controlled trial performed in 273 individuals, daily treatment with folic acid (2 mg), vitamin B6 (25 mg), and vitamin B12 (0.5 mg) for approximately 7 years suggested that this combination of vitamins might be an effective, safe, and affordable intervention to reduce the risk of depression after stroke (Almeida et al., 2010).

A recent study found no strong evidence that folic acid supplementation reduced the risk of depression during pregnancy and up to 8 months after pregnancy. However, this work found evidence to suggest that folic acid supplements during pregnancy protected against depression 21 months postpartum (Lewis et al., 2011).

Considering the following findings: a) depressive patients frequently have a functional folic acid deficiency (which can be related to high homocysteine levels) and poor response to antidepressant therapy (Coppen and Bailey, 2000; Papakostas et al., 2004a; 2005); b) folic acid is associated with the synthesis of monoamines (Stahl, 2007); c) folic acid supplementation can potentiate the effects of antidepressant medication (Resler et al., 2008; Almeida et al., 2010; Christensen et al., 2011); it is reasonable to conclude that this vitamin can be a safe, simple and cheap alternative for the treatment of depression (Roberts et al., 2007). In support of this hypothesis, it has been shown that folic acid supplementation increases medication response in depressive patients (Fava, 2010; Fava and Mischoulon, 2010; Nahas and Sheikh, 2011), probably due to an increase in the availability of monoamines (Stahl, 2007).

Considering that several clinical findings indicate a strong correlation between folic acid and depression, some preclinical studies have emerged to elucidate the possible antidepressant effect of this vitamin in animal model of depression, as reviewed in Table 2. The antidepressant potential of folic acid (administered either through the oral, intracerebroventricular, or intraperitoneal route) was investigated in mice that were submitted to the forced swimming and the tail suspension tests, two behavioral tests that are predictive of antidepressant activity (Brocardo et al., 2008a). In these tests, a reduction in immobility time is the parameter used to infer the antidepressant-like action of drugs (Porsolt et al., 1977; Steru et al., 1985).

Table 1. Summary of findings from clinical studies evaluating the role of folic acid in depression

Study	Major Findings
Carney, 1967	Patients suffering from various psychiatric syndromes had low serum folic acid concentrations.
Reynolds et al., 1970	24% of depressed patients had low serum folic acid concentrations.
Carney and Sheffield, 1978	21.3% of 272 psychiatric patients had low serum folic acid levels.
Ghadirian et al., 1980	Low folic acid content in depressive patients was correlated with higher scores on the Hamilton Rating Scale (HDRS) for depression.
Botez et al., 1982	Folic acid supplementation enhanced 5-hydroxyindoleacetic in the cerebrospinal fluid (CSF) of psychiatric patients with folic acid deficiency.
Botez et al., 1984	Folic acid supplementation (10 mg daily) improved the scores on Ottawa-Wechsler Scale in psychiatric patients with serum and CSF folic acid deficiency.
Abou-Saleh and Coppen, 1989	Depressive patients had low serum and red blood cell (RBC) folic acid content.
Levitt and Joffe, 1989	Duration of depressive episode was significantly correlated with low folic acid levels.
Carney, 1990	Depressive patients had RBC folic acid deficiency (below 200 μg/l).
Godfrey et al., 1990	33% of 123 patients with psychiatric disorders including depression had low RBC folic acid status and the supplementation with methylfolate (15 mg/day, for 6 months) improved clinical and social recovery.
Passeri et al., 1993	5'-Methyltetrahydrofolic acid (5'-MTHF) supplementation reduced the HDRS score in depressed patients with borderline or definite folic acid deficiency and in normofolatemic patients after 3 weeks of treatment.
Wesson et al., 1994	Increased RBC folic acid levels was associated with a lower severity of depression and a better response to desmethylimipramine in depressive patients.
Arinami et al., 1997	The T677 allele of the methylenetetrahydrofolate reductase (MTHFR) gene was associated with schizophrenia and depression.
Fava et al., 1997	Depressive patients with low folic acid level were more susceptible to developing melancholic depression and less prone to respond to treatment with fluoxetine.
Herran et al., 1999	Depressive patients had serum folic acid deficiency but normal RBC folic acid.
Bottiglieri et al., 2000	52% of depressed patients had significant low serum, RBC, and CSF folic acid content.
Lindeman et al., 2000	Folic acid deficiency was associated with cognitive dysfunction and depression.
Coppen and Bailey, 2000	Folic acid supplementation (500 μg/day) combined with fluoxetine (20 mg/day) improved the antidepressant effect of fluoxetine, particularly in women.

Study	Major Findings
Alpert et al., 2002	An eight-week open study showed that folinic acid (an active form of folic acid, 15 to 30 mg/day for eight weeks) enhanced the effects of selective serotonin reuptake inhibitor-refractory depression.
Tolmunen et al., 2003	Patients with low intake of folic acid had elevated depressive symptoms.
Kelly et al., 2004	Patients with MTHFR C677T genotype had an increased risk for developing depressive episodes.
Papakostas et al., 2004a	Depressive patients with low folic acid status were associated with poorer response to treatment with fluoxetine.
Papakostas et al., 2004b	Depressive patients with low folic acid status were associated with relapse during continuation treatment with fluoxetine.
Papakostas et al., 2005	Depressive patients with low folic acid status were associated with delay to start the improvement of psychiatric symptoms during treatment with fluoxetine.
Williams et al., 2005	Folic acid supplementation (100 mg for 6 weeks followed by 200 mg for 6 weeks) did not improve psychiatric symptoms associated with depression.
Lewis et al., 2006	A meta-analysis showed that polymorphism (C677T) in MTHFR was associated with the risk of depression.
Roberts et al., 2007	Folic acid supplementation augmented antidepressant response.
Astorg et al., 2008	Low intake of folic acid predisposed recurrent depressive episodes in men.
Kendrick et al., 2008	Low RBC folic acid content did not predict the incidence of depressive symptoms.
Ford et al., 2008	Folic acid supplementation was not effective in reducing depressive symptoms.
Resler et al., 2008	Folic acid supplementation combined with fluoxetine significantly reduced the HDRS scores in depressive patients.
Almeida et al., 2010	Supplementation with folic acid, as well as vitamins B6 and B12 in post-stroke survivors reduced the risk to depressive episodes.
Nanri et al., 2010	A higher serum folic acid status decreased the prevalence of depressive symptoms in men.
Skarupski et al., 2010	Folic acid supplementation was not effective in reducing depressive symptoms in depressed patients.
Walker et al., 2010	Folic acid supplementation was not effective in reducing depressive symptoms.
Christensen et al., 2011	Folic acid plus vitamin B12 supplementation improved depressive symptoms.
Fathy et al., 2011	33% of patients with depressive disorder or anxiety had MTFR C677T polymorphism. Additionally, there was a negative correlation between the severity of depression and folic acid status in depressive patients.
Lewis et al., 2011	Folic acid supplements during pregnancy protected against depression 21 months postpartum

Moreover, in this study, Brocardo et al. (2008a) also used pharmacological tools to investigate the involvement of the serotonergic and noradrenergic systems in mediating the antidepressant-like effect of folic acid. The results of this study support the notion that the anti-depressant effects of folic acid might result from the activation of both serotonergic (5-HT_{1A} and 5-$HT_{2A/2C}$ receptors) and noradrenergic (α_1- and α_2-adrenoceptors) systems (Brocardo et al., 2008a). Furthermore, the antidepressant-like effects of this vitamin were shown to be dependent on the inhibition of either *N*-methyl-D-aspartate (NMDA) receptors or nitric oxide (NO) and cyclic guonosine monophosphate (cGMP) synthesis (Brocardo et al., 2008b), as well as through an interaction with the opioid system (μ_1 and δ receptors) (Brocardo et al., 2009). It is also important to emphasize that co-administration of sub-effective doses of folic acid and fluoxetine in mice produced antidepressant-like effects as assessed with the forced swimming test (Brocardo et al., 2008a). Moreover, using the same behavioral assessment tool, it was possible to verify that folic acid alone or combined with estradiol or fluoxetine also has antidepressant-like effects in ovariectomized female rats (Molina-Hernández et al., 2011). Furthermore, it was recently reported that the antidepressant effect of folic acid might also be dependent, at least in part, on the inhibition of glycogen synthase kinase-3 (GSK-3β) and activation of peroxisome proliferator-activated receptor-γ (PPARγ) (Budni et al., 2011).

Although these studies clearly indicate that folic acid plays an important role in depression, the exact mechanisms of this relationship remain to be fully elucidated. Furthermore, future well-designed and adequately powered clinical trials are warranted in order to ascertain the prophylactic and therapeutic properties of folic acid, including its appropriate formulation, optimal dose, and ideal duration of treatment.

Folic Acid and Bipolar Disorder

Bipolar disorder is a psychiatric disease characterized by mood alterations that are associated with recurrent depression and mania throughout lifetime (Swann, 2005). Mania is the most specific manifestation of bipolar disorder and is defined by an abnormally elevated mood state characterized by such symptoms as inappropriate elation, increased irritability, severe insomnia, grandiose notions, increased speed and/or volume of speech, disconnected and racing thoughts, increased sexual desire, markedly increased energy and activity level, poor judgment, and inappropriate social behavior (Berrios, 2004). Early studies have shown that folic acid deficiency is associated with a number of neurological and psychiatric disorders, including bipolar disorder (Hasanah et al., 1997; Ozbek et al., 2008).

Since monoamines are involved in mood regulation (Elhwuegi, 2004) and serotonin has been shown to contribute to mania (Shiah and Yatham, 2000), it is possible that bipolar patients have an increased need for folic acid (Coppen et al., 1986). In addition, several studies have also observed disturbances of homocysteine metabolism in bipolar disorder (Osher et al., 2004; Dittmann et al., 2007; 2008). Moreover, both genetic polymorphisms that alter enzymes involved in the metabolism of homocysteine such as MTHFR and folic acid deficiency, which can result in variations in the levels of homocysteine (Jacques et al., 1996), have been correlated with bipolar disorder. Indeed, Ozbek et al. (2008) investigated the effect of polymorphic variants of MTHFR (c.1298A>C and c.677C>T) on homocysteine, folic acid, and vitamin B12 levels in 197 bipolar patients, 278 unaffected first-degree relatives, and 238 normal controls and found that homocysteine levels are higher and folic acid levels are lower in patients with bipolar disorder as compared with the healthy controls.

Table 2. Summary of findings from preclinical studies that document the antidepressant-like effect of folic acid

Study	Major Findings
Brocardo et al., 2008a	Folic acid had antidepressant-like effects in mice as assessed in the FST and TST. This effect involves serotonergic (5-HT_{1A} and 5-$HT_{2A/2C}$ receptors) and noradrenergic (α_1- and α_2-adrenoceptors) systems.
Brocardo et al., 2008b	The antidepressant-like effects of folic acid involve NMDA receptors and modulation of the L-arginine-NO-cGMP pathway.
Brocardo et al., 2009	The antidepressant-like effects of folic acid involve δ- and μ-opioid receptors.
Molina-Hernández et al., 2011	Folic acid alone or combined with estradiol or fluoxetine has antidepressant-like effects in ovariectomized female rats as assessed in the FST.
Budni et al., 2011	The antidepressant-like effects of folic acid involve inhibition of GSK-3β and activation of PPARγ.

Hyperhomocysteinaemia may also play a role in the pathophysiology of neurocognitive deficits in bipolar disorder, with a higher impact in older patients or in patients who had delayed onset of illness (Osher et al., 2004; Dittmann et al., 2007; 2008). Osher et al. (2004) measured homocysteine levels in 41 euthymic outpatients with bipolar disorder and compared them with 305 subjects from a large employee health-screening program. They found that bipolar patients who show functional deterioration have elevated plasma levels of homocysteine as compared with control individuals. Dittmann et al. (2007) used neuropsychological tests in 55 euthymic bipolar patients and 17 healthy controls and observed an association between neuropsychological measures and elevated homocysteine levels in euthymic bipolar patients. In addition, a study was conducted between 2002 and 2006 in 75 euthymic bipolar patients and 42 healthy controls in order to investigate the potential relationship of elevated homocysteine levels and cognitive impairment in bipolar patients. In agreement with the previous studies, this trial also found an association between homocysteine levels and verbal learning, delayed memory, as well as executive function in the patient group (Dittmann et al., 2008).

In agreement with these clinical studies, we have recently shown that folic acid can prevent biochemical and behavioral alterations in an ouabain-induced animal model of mania in rats (Brocardo et al., 2010). In addition, other clinical studies have shown reduced folic acid levels in erythrocytes (Hasanah et al., 1997) and serum (Ozbek et al., 2008) of manic patients, demonstrating that folic acid may play an important role during the manic phase of bipolar disorder. Furthermore, it has been reported that folic acid can enhance the prophylactic effects of lithium on affective morbidity (Coppen and Abou-Saleh, 1982; Coppen et al., 1986). A recent clinical study has also shown that folic acid can be an effective adjuvant to sodium valproate in the treatment of the acute phase of mania in patients with bipolar disorder (Behzadi et al., 2009). A summary of the main findings are provided below in Table 3.

Taken together, these studies strongly indicate that folic acid can be a putative candidate for the treatment of bipolar disorder. Further preclinical and clinical studies are thus warranted in order to confirm this hypothesis and to investigate whether folic acid treatment has beneficial effects in patients with normal folic acid levels as well as in individuals with folic acid deficiency.

Table 3. Summary of findings from preclinical and clinical studies that investigated the role of folic acid in bipolar disorders

Study	Major Findings
Brocardo et al., 2010	Folic acid demonstrated antimanic-like effects in the animal model of mania induced by ouabain in rats.
Coppen and Abou-Saleh, 1982	Folic acid combined with lithium decreased affective morbidity.
Coppen et al., 1986	Folic acid enhanced the prophylactic effects of lithium on affective morbidity.
Hasanah et al., 1997	Reduced folate levels in erythrocytes of bipolar patients.
Ozbek et al., 2008	Folate levels were lower and homocysteine levels were higher in the serum of bipolar patients.
Behzadi et al., 2009	Folic acid was an effective adjuvant to sodium valproate in the treatment of the acute phase of mania.

Folic Acid and Schizophrenia

Schizophrenia is a complex psychiatric disease that is believed to result from multiple genetic and environmental factors (Levi and Waxman, 1975; Miyamoto et al., 2003). This disease is often described in terms of positive and negative symptoms. Positive symptoms can include delusions, disordered thoughts and speech, as well as tactile, auditory, visual, olfactory and gustatory hallucinations, typically regarded as manifestations of psychosis (Frith and Done, 1989). Negative symptoms are deficits of normal emotional responses or of other thought processes such as poverty of speech, impoverished ability to express emotion, lack of motivation, and apathy (Rummel et al., 2005). While antipsychotic drugs are very effective for the positive symptoms of schizophrenia, the treatment of negative symptoms is still a major problem (Crow, 1980; Andreasen, 1985).

Studies on the association of folic acid deficiency with schizophrenia (summarized in Table 4) extend back to the mid 1960's (Krebs et al., 2009). Carney (1967) found an incidence of folic acid deficiency in a group of 423 psychiatric patients. This study established that a high incidence (20%) of folic acid deficiency occurs in patients with schizophrenia. In agreement, a study conducted on 243 psychiatric patients indicated that schizophrenic patients had red cell folic acid deficiency (below 200 μg/l) (Carney, 1990). However, a recent study by García-Miss et al. (2010) observed low levels of folic acid in RBC and increased levels of TNF-α, interleucyne-6 and homocysteine. It is believed that folic acid treatment in patients with hyperhomocysteinemia reduces the release of both homocysteine and proinflammatory cytokines from monocytes (Wang et al., 2005). However, folic acid treatment decreased not only the levels of homocysteine, but also the inflammatory response in schizophrenic patients (García-Miss et al., 2010). Furthermore, another recent study showed that deficiency of folic acid both in the serum and RBC is common in schizophrenic patients, suggesting that decreased levels of folic acid in the plasma may act as a risk factor for schizophrenia (Saedisomeolia et al., 2011). These findings corroborate the study by Kale et al. (2010) that showed significantly lower levels of folic acid and vitamin B12 in the plasma and of folic acid in RBC as well as a significant increase in plasma homocysteine and cortisol levels in schizophrenic patients. Moreover, a case reported by Ho et al. (2010) showed that a 13-year-old previously healthy subject with schizophrenic symptoms and progressively worsening catatonia had cerebral folic acid deficiency and elevated titers of folic acid receptor-blocking antibodies, indicating that folic acid deficiency may be related with catatonic schizophrenia.

Individuals with schizophrenia and low serum levels of folic acid are especially vulnerable to the negative symptoms of this disease, since serum folic acid concentration appears to be inversely correlated with the severity of negative symptoms on the Scale for Assessment of Negative Symptoms (Goff et al., 2004). These findings corroborate a similar study that examined the incidence of folic acid deficiency, based on serum determinations, in relation to the severity of negative symptoms in schizophrenic patients (Herran et al., 1999).

Several studies indicate that prenatal deficiencies of certain micronutrients, including folic acid, may play an important role in schizophrenia (Brown et al., 1996; Susser et al., 1996; Hoek et al., 1998; McGrath et al., 2011), and folic acid deficiency during early pregnancy has been hypothesized as a cause of schizophrenia in the offspring (Smits and Essed, 2001; Smits et al., 2004; McGrath et al., 2011). Postpartum restoration of folic acid levels to normal status may take up to 1 year (Smith et al., 1983; Açkurt et al., 1995; Bruinse and Van den Berg, 1995). Accordingly, the risk of developing schizophrenia may be elevated for children conceived within this restorative period (Smits et al., 2004).

Table 4. Summary of findings from clinical studies evaluating the involvement of folic acid in schizophrenia

Study	Major Findings
Carney, 1967	Patients suffering from various psychiatric syndromes had low serum folic acid concentrations.
Carney, 1990	Schizophrenic patients had RBC folic acid deficiency (below 200 μg/l).
Godfrey, 1990	33% of 123 patients with psychiatric disorders including schizophrenia had low RBC folic acid content and supplementation with methylfolate (15 mg/day, for 6 months) improved clinical and social recovery.
Herran et al., 1999	Schizophrenic patients had serum folic acid deficiency but normal RBC folic acid.
Smits and Essed, 2001 Smits et al., 2004	Patients conceived shortly after another birth (during maternal folic acid deficiency) had an increased risk for schizophrenia.
Muntjewerff et al., 2003	Schizophrenic patients had low plasma folic acid status and high RBC folic acid concentration. MTFR C677T polymorphism was not associated with an increased risk for schizophrenia.
Goff et al., 2004	Schizophrenic patients had low serum folic acid concentration, which was inversely correlated with the Scale for Assessment of Negative Symptoms total score.
Smits et al., 2004	Patients conceived shortly after another birth (during maternal folic acid deficiency) had an increased risk for schizophrenia.
Muntjewerff et al., 2005	A meta-analysis showed that folic acid deficiency is associated to risk of schizophrenia.
Muntjewerff et al., 2006	A meta-analysis showed that MTHFR 677C>T polymorphism is associated to risk of schizophrenia.
Haidemenos et al., 2007 Petronijevic et al., 2008	Schizophrenia was not associated with folic acid deficiency.
Roffman et al., 2008	MTHFR 677C>T polymorphism was associated with the severity of negative symptoms in schizophrenic patients.
García-Miss et al., 2010	Schizophrenic patients had low RBC folic acid levels and elevated homocysteine, interleukin-6 (IL-6), and tumor necrosis factor-alpha (TNF-α) levels. MTHFR 677C>T polymorphism was not associated with the risk for schizophrenia.
Ho et al., 2010	A case study showed that a schizophrenic teenager with cerebral folic acid deficiency had catatonic symptoms.
Kale et al., 2010	Significantly low plasma and RBC folic acid and vitamin B12 concentrations were observed in schizophrenic patients.
Yoshimi et al., 2010	MTHFR 677C>T polymorphism was associated with the severity of negative symptoms in schizophrenic patients.
Saedisomeolia et al., 2011	Significantly low serum and RBC folic acid content was observed in schizophrenic patients.

However, although all evidence indicating that folic acid deficiency is a risk factor for schizophrenia, there are recent reports that contradict this view (Haidemenos et al., 2007; Petronijevic et al., 2008). For example, an increase in folic acid content in RBC of schizophrenic patients has been documented (Muntjewerff et al., 2003).

Surprisingly, despite numerous reports on the association between folic acid deficiency and schizophrenia, there are relatively few controlled clinical trials that have tested the potential beneficial effect of folic acid supplementation on this disorder (Godfrey et al., 1990; Levine et al., 2006). Godfrey et al. (1990) showed that methylfolate supplementation significantly improved clinical and social recovery among both depressed and schizophrenic patients in a double-blind, placebo-controlled trial. Additionally, another double-blind placebo-controlled trial of methylfolate was performed.

The administration of this compound (15 mg/day) for 6 months resulted in the attenuation of the psychiatric symptoms of schizophrenia (Godfrey et al., 1990). In a placebo-controlled cross-over trial of 42 schizophrenic patients with elevated serum homocysteine levels, Levine et al. (2006) reported a significantly reduction in the total scores of the Positive and Negative Syndrome Scale in the group who received folic acid and vitamin B12 for 3 months.

Both hyperhomocysteinemia and polymorphisms in MTHFR, encoding a critical enzyme for the metabolism of both folic acid and homocysteine have been linked to schizophrenia (Muntjewerff et al., 2005; Muntjewerff et al., 2006; Yoshimi et al., 2010) and strong epidemiological evidence supports this relationship (Allen et al., 2008). Additionally, 677T allele load is associated with the severity of the negative symptoms in schizophrenic patients (Roffman et al., 2008). From a clinical point of view, it is interesting to note that homocysteine-reducing strategies improve psychopathology in chronic schizophrenic patients with hyperhomocysteinemia (Levine et al., 2006). Moreover, Brown et al. (2007) found that elevated third trimester homocysteine levels (caused by low folic acid levels) were associated with a 2-fold increase in the risk of developing adult schizophrenia. However, despite the evidence pointing towards an association between MTHFR C667T mutation and schizophrenia, there is a recent report that contradicts this idea (García-Miss et al., 2010), indicating that further studies are required in order to clarify this hypothesis.

Conclusion

Basic research and clinical studies have shown that folic acid plays a role in the pathophysiology and/or treatment of psychiatric disorders such as depression, bipolar disorder and schizophrenia. Regarding this issue, the majority of the studies published to date deal with the effects of folic acid deficiency/supplementation on depressive symptoms, indicating that the potential of this vitamin as an antidepressant drug should be further evaluated. The studies involving the relationship between the levels of folic acid and bipolar disorder are scarce and the possible role of this vitamin in the schizophrenia is not well established. Thus, we conclude that further experimental evidence is warranted in order to ascertain the involvement of folic acid in the pathophysiology and treatment of these psychiatric diseases.

Acknowledgments

Authors thank Joana Gil-Mohapel (Ph.D., Division of Medical Sciences, Island Medical Program, University of Victoria, Victoria, BC, Canada) for revising the chapter.

References

Abou-Saleh, MT; Coppen, A. Serum and red blood cell folate in depression. *Acta Psychiatr. Scand.,* 1989 80(1), 78-82.

Açkurt, F; Wetherilt, H; Löker, M; Hacibekirog, M. Biochemical assessment of nutritional status in pre- and post-natal Turkish women and outcome of pregnancy. *Eur. J. Clin. Nutr.,* 1995 49, 613-622.

Allen, NC; Bagade, S; McQueen, MB; Ioannidis, JP; Kavvoura, FK; Khoury, MJ; Tanzi, RE; Bertram, L. Systematic meta-analyses and field synopsis of genetic association studies in schizophrenia: the SzGene database. *Nat. Genet.,* 2008 40, 827-834.

Almeida, OP; Marsh, K; Alfonso, H; Flicker, L; Davis, TM; Hankey, GJ. B-vitamins reduce the long-term risk of depression after stroke: The VITATOPS-DEP trial. *Ann. Neurol.*, 2010 68(4), 503-510.

Alpert, JE; Mischoulon, D; Rubenstein, GE; Bottonari, K; Nierenberg, AA; Fava, M. Folinic acid (Leucovorin) as an adjunctive treatment for SSRI-refractory depression. *Ann. Clin. Psychiatry,* 2002 14(1), 33-38.

Andreasen, NC. Positive vs. negative schizophrenia: a critical evaluation. *Schizophr. Bull.,* 1985 11, 380-389.

Arinami, T; Yamada, N; Yamakawa-Kobayashi, K; Hamaguchi, H; Toru, M. Methylenetetrahydrofolate reductase variant and schizophrenia/ depression. *Am. J. Med. Genet.,* 1997 74(5), 526-528.

Astorg, P; Couthouis, A; de Courcy, GP; Bertrais, S; Arnault, N; Meneton, P; Galan, P; Hercberg, S. Association of folate intake with the occurrence of depressive episodes in middle-aged French men and women. *Br. J. Nutr.,* 2008 100(1), 183-187.

Behzadi, AH; Omrani, Z; Chalian, M; Asadi, S; Ghadiri, M. Folic acid efficacy as an alternative drug added to sodium valproate in the treatment of acute phase of mania in bipolar disorder: a double-blind randomized controlled trial. *Acta Psychiatr. Scand.,* 2009 120, 441-445.

Berrios, GE. Of Mania: introduction (Classic text no. 57). *Hist. Psychiatry*, 2004 15, 105-124.

Botez, MI; Young, SN; Bachevalier, J; Gauthier, S. Effect of folic acid and vitamin B12 deficiencies on 5-hydroxyindoleacetic acid in human cerebrospinal fluid. *Ann. Neurol.*, 1982 12(5), 479-484.

Botez, MI; Botez, T; Maag, U. The Wechsler subtests in mild organic brain damage associated with folate deficiency. *Psychol. Med.*, 1984 14(2), 431-437.

Bottiglieri, T; Laundy, M; Crellin, R; Toone, B; Carney, M; Reynolds E. Homocysteine, folate, methylation, and monoamine metabolism in depression. *J. Neurol. Neurosurg. Psychiatry*, 2000 69(2), 228-232.

Brocardo, PS; Budni, J; Kaster, MP; Santos, ARS; Rodrigues, ALS. Folic acid administration produces an antidepressant-like effect in mice: evidence for the involvement of the serotonergic and noradrenergic systems. *Neuropharmacology*, 2008a 54, 464-473.

Brocardo, OS; Budni, J; Lobato, KR; Kaster, MP; Rodrigues, ALS. Antidepressant-like effect of folic acid: Involvement of NMDA receptors and L-arginine-nitric oxide-cyclic guanosine monophosphate pathway. *Eur. J. Pharmacol.*, 2008b 598, 37-42.

Brocardo, PS; Budni, J; Lobato, KR; Santos, ARS, Rodrigues, ALS. Evidence for the involvement of the opioid system in the antidepressant-like effect of folic acid in the mouse forced swimming test. *Behav. Brain Res.*, 2009 200, 122-127.

Brocardo, OS; Budni, J; Pavesi, E; Franco, JL; Uliano-Silva, M; Trevisan, R; Terenzi, MG; Dafre, AL; Rodrigues, AL. Folic acid administration prevents ouabain-induced hyperlocomotion and alterations in oxidative stress markers in the rat brain. *Bipolar. Disord.*, 2010 12, 414-424.

Brown, AS; Susser, ES; Butler, PD; Andrews, RR; Kaufmann, CA; Gorman, JM. Neurobiological plausibility of prenatal nutritional deprivation as a risk factor for schizophrenia. *J. Nerv. Ment. Dis.*, 1996 184, 71- 85.

Brown, AS; Bottiglieri, T; Schaefer, CA; Quesenberry, CP Jr; Liu, L; Bresnahan, M; Susser, ES. Elevated prenatal homocysteine levels as a risk factor for schizophrenia. *Arch. Gen. Psychiatry*, 2007 64, 31-39.

Bruinse, HW; Van den Berg, H. Changes of some vitamin levels during and after normal pregnancy. *Eur. J. Obstet. Gynecol. Reprod. Biol.*, 1995 61, 31-37.

Budni, J; Lobato, KR; Binfaré, RW; Freitas, AE; Costa, AP; Saavedra, MDM; Leal, RB; Lopez, MG; Rodrigues, ALS. Involvement of PI3K, GSK-3β and PPARγ in the antidepressant-like effect of folic acid in the forced swimming test in mice. *J. Psychopharmacol.*, 2011, *in press*.

Carney, MW. Serum folate values in 423 psychiatric patients. *Br. Med. J.*, 1967 4(5578), 512-516.

Carney, MW; Sheffield, BF. Serum folic acid and B12 in 272 psychiatric in-patients. *Psychol. Med.*, 1978 8(1),139-144.

Carney, MW; Chary, TK; Laundy, M; Bottiglieri, T; Chanarin, I; Reynolds, EH; Toone, B. Red cell folate concentrations in psychiatric patients. *J. Affect. Disord.*, 1990 19, 207-213.

Christensen, H; Aiken, A; Batterham, PJ; Walker, J; Mackinnon, AJ; Fenech, M; Hickie, IB. No clear potentiation of antidepressant medication effects by folic acid+vitamin B(12) in a large community sample. *J. Affect. Disord.*, 2011 130(1-2), 37-45.

Coppen, A; Abou-Saleh, MT. Plasma folate and affective morbidity during long-term lithium therapy. *Br. J. Psychiatry*, 1982 141, 87-89.

Coppen, A; Chaudhry, S; Swade, C. Folic acid enhances lithium prophylaxis. *J. Affect. Disord.*, 1986 10, 9-13.

Coppen, A; Bailey J. Enhancement of the antidepressant action of fluoxetine by folic acid: a randomised, placebo controlled trial. *J. Affect. Disord*, 2000 60(2), 121-130.

Coppen, A; Bolander-Gouaille, C. Treatment of depression: time to consider folic acid and vitamin B12. *J. Psychopharmacol.*, 2005 19(1), 59-65.

Crow, TJ. Molecular pathology of schizophrenia: more than one disease process? *Br. Med. J.*, 1980 280, 66-68.

Dittmann, S; Seemuller, F; Schwarz, MJ; Kleindienst, N; Stampfer, R; Zach, J; Born, C; Bernhard, B; Fast, K; Grunze, H; Engel, RR; Severus, E. Association of cognitive deficits with elevated homocysteine levels in euthymic bipolar patients and its impact on psychosocial functioning: preliminary results. *Bipolar. Disord.*, 2007 9, 63-70.

Dittmann, S; Seemuller, F; Grunze, HC; Schwarz, MJ; Zach, J; Fast, K; Born, C; Dargel, S; Engel, RR; Bernhard, B; Moller, HJ; Riedel, M; Severus, WE. The impact of homocysteine levels on cognition in euthymic bipolar patients: a cross-sectional study. *J. Clin. Psychiatry*, 2008 69, 899-906.

Elhwuegi, AS. Central monoamines and their role in major depression. *Prog. Neuropsychopharmacol. Biol. Psychiatry*, 2004 28, 435-451.

Fathy, H; Abd, E; Sherine, M; Abdou, H; Adel A; Abdou A. Methyltetrahydrofolate reductase polymorphism, folic acid, and B12 in a sample of patients with depressive and anxiety symptoms. *Middle East Current Psychiatry,* 2011 18, 118-125.

Fava, M; Borus, JS; Alpert, JE; Nierenberg, AA; Rosenbaum, JF; Bottiglieri, T. Folate, vitamin B12, and homocysteine in major depressive disorder. *Am. J. Psychiatry*, 1997 154(3), 426-428.

Fava, M. Using complementary and alternative medicines for depression. *J. Clin. Psychiatry*, 2010 71(9), e24.

Fava, M; Mischoulon, D. Evidence for folate in combination with antidepressants at initiation of therapy. *J. Clin. Psychiatry*, 2010 71(11), e3.

Farah, A. The role of L-methylfolate in depressive disorders. *CNS Spectr.*, 2009 14(2), 2-7.

Ford, A; Flicker, L; Thomas, J; Norman, P; Jamrozik, K; Almeida, O. Vitamins B12, B6, and folic acid for onset of depressive symptoms in older men: results from a 2-year placebo-controlled randomized trial. *J. Clin. Psychiatry,* 2008 69(8), 1203-1209.

Frith, C; Done, J. Positive symptoms of schizophrenia. *Br. J. Psychiatry*, 1989 154, 569-570.

García-Miss, M del R; Pérez-Mutul, J; López-Canul, B; Solís-Rodríguez, F; Puga-Machado, L; Oxté-Cabrera, A; Gurubel-Maldonado, J; Arankowsky-Sandoval, G. Folate, homocysteine, interleukin-6, and tumor necrosis factor alfa levels, but not the methylenetetrahydrofolate reductase C677T polymorphism, are risk factors for schizophrenia. *J. Psychiatr. Res.*, 2010 44(7), 441-446.

Ghadirian, AM; Ananth, J; Engelsmann, F. Folic acid deficiency and depression. *Psychosomatics*, 1980 21(11), 926-929.

Godfrey, PS; Toone, BK; Carney, MW; Flynn, TG; Bottiglieri, T; Laundy, M; Chanarin, I; Reynolds EH. Enhancement of recovery from psychiatric illness by methylfolate. *Lancet*, 1990 336(8712), 392-395.

Goff, DC; Bottiglieri, T; Arning, E; Shih, V; Freudenreich, O; Evins, AE; Henderson, DC; Baer, L; Coyle, J. Folate, homocysteine, and negative symptoms in schizophrenia. *Am. J. Psychiatry*, 2004 161, 1705-1708.

Haidemenos, A; Kontis, D; Gazi, A; Kallai, E; Allin, M; Lucia, B. Plasma homocysteine, folate and B12 in chronic schizophrenia. *Prog. Neuropsychopharmacol. Biol. Psychiatry*, 2007 31(6), 1289 1296.

Hasanah, CI; Khan, UA; Musalmah, M; Razali, SM. Reduced red-cell folate in mania. *J. Affect. Disord.*, 1997 46(2), 95-99.

Herrán, A; García-Unzueta, MT; Amado, JÁ; López-Cordovilla, JJ; Díez-Manrique, JF; Vázquez-Barquero, JL. Folate levels in psychiatric outpatients. *Psychiatry Clin. Neurosci.*, 1999 53, 531-533.

Herbert, V. Experimental nutritional folate deficiency in man. *Trans Assoc. Am. Physicians*, 1962 75, 307-320.

Ho, A; Michelson, D; Aaen, G; Ashwal, S. Cerebral folate deficiency presenting as adolescent catatonic schizophrenia: a case report. *J. Child Neurol.*, 2010 25(7), 898-900.

Hoek, HW; Brown, AS; Susser, E. The Dutch famine and schizophrenia spectrum disorders. *Soc. Psychiatry Psychiatr. Epidemiol.*, 1998 33, 373-379.

Jacques, PF; Bostom, AG; Williams, RR; Ellison, RC; Eckfeldt, JH; Rosenberg, IH; Selhub, J; Rozen, R. Relation between folate status, a common mutation in methylenetetrahydrofolate reductase, and plasma homocysteine concentrations. *Circulation*, 1996 93(1), 7-9.

Kale, A; Naphade, N; Sapkale, S; Kamaraju, M; Pillai, A; Joshi, S; Mahadik, S. Reduced folic acid, vitamin B12 and docosahexaenoic acid and increased homocysteine and cortisol in never-medicated schizophrenia patients: implications for altered one-carbon metabolism. *Psychiatry Res.*, 2010 175(1-2), 47-53.

Kelly, CB; McDonnell, AP; Johnston, TG; Mulholland, C; Cooper, SJ; McMaster, D; Evans, A; Whitehead, AS. The MTHFR C677T polymorphism is associated with depressive episodes in patients from Northern Ireland. *J. Psychopharmacol.*, 2004 18(4), 567-571.

Kendrick, T; Dunn, N; Robinson, S; Oestmann, A; Godfrey, K; Cooper, C; Inskip, H. Southampton Women's Survey Study Group. A longitudinal study of blood folate levels and depressive symptoms among young women in the Southampton Women's Survey. *J. Epidemiol. Community Health*, 2008 62(11), 966-972.

Kessler, RC; Berglund, P; Demler, O; Jin, R; Merikangas, KR; Walters, EE. Lifetime prevalence and age-of-onset distributions of DSM-IV disorders in the National Comorbidity Survey Replication. *Arch. Gen. Psychiatry* 2005 62, 593-602.

Khanna, S; Kapoor, P; Pillai, KK; Vohora, D. Homocysteine in neurological disease: a marker or a cause? *CNS Neurol. Disord. Drug Targets*, 2011 10(3), 361-369.

Krebs, MO; Bellon, A; Mainguy, G; Jay, TM; Frieling, H. One-carbon metabolism and schizophrenia: current challenges and future directions. *Trends Mol. Med.*, 2009 15(12), 562-570.

Krishnan, V; Nestler, EJ. Linking molecules to mood: new insight into the biology of depression. *Am. J. Psychiatry*, 2010 167(11), 1305-1320.

Kronenberg, G; Colla, M; Endres, M. Folic acid, neurodegenerative and neuropsychiatric disease. *Curr. Mol. Med.*, 2009 9(3), 315-323.

Kruman, II; Culmsee, C; Chan, SL; Kruman, Y; Guo, Z; Penix, L; Mattson, MP. Homocysteine elicits a DNA damage response in neurons that promotes apoptosis and hypersensitivity to excitotoxicity. *J. Neurosci.*, 2000 20, 6920-6926.

Lazarou, C; Kapsou, M. The role of folic acid in prevention and treatment of depression: an overview of existing evidence and implications for practice. *Complement. Ther. Clin. Pract.*, 2010 16(3), 161-166.

Lee, S; Jeong, J; Kwak, Y; Park, SK. Depression research: where are we now? *Mol. Brain.,* 2010 3, 8.

Levi, RN; Waxman, S. Schizophrenia, epilepsy, cancer, methionine, and folate metabolism. Pathogenesis of schizophrenia. *Lancet*, 1975 2, 11-13.

Levine, J; Stahl, Z; Sela, BA; Ruderman, V; Shumaico, O; Babushkin, I; Osher, Y; Bersudsky, Y; Belmaker, RH. Homocysteine-reducing strategies improve symptoms in chronic schizophrenic patients with hyperhomocysteinemia. *Biol. Psychiatry*, 2006 60, 265-269.

Levitt, AJ; Joffe, RT. Folate, B12 and life course of depressive illness. *Biol. Psychiatry*, 1989 25, 867-872.

Lewis, SJ; Lawlor, DA; Davey Smith, G; Araya, R; Timpson, N; Day, INM; Ebrahim, S. The thermolabile variant of MTHFR is associated with depression in the British Women's Heart and Health Study and a meta-analysis. *Mol. Psychiatry*, 2006 11 352-360.

Lewis SJ, Araya R, Leary S, Smith GD, Ness A. Folic acid supplementation during pregnancy may protect against depression 21 months after pregnancy, an effect modified by MTHFR C677T genotype. *Eur. J. Clin. Nutr.*, 2011, *in press*. doi: 10.1038/ejcn.2011.136.

Lindeman, RD; Romero, LJ; Koehler, KM; Liang, HC; LaRue, A; Baumgartner, RN; Garry, PJ. Serum vitamin B12, C and folate concentrations in the New Mexico elder health survey: correlations with cognitive and affective functions. *J. Am. Coll. Nutr.*, 200 19(1), 68-76.

Lipton, SA; Kim, WK; Choi, YB; Kumar, S; D'Emilia, DM; Rayudu, PV; Arnelle, DR; Stamler, JS. Neurotoxicity associated with dual actions of homocysteine at the N-methyl-D-aspartate receptor. *Proc. Natl. Acad. Sci. USA*, 1997 94, 5923-5928.

Lucock, M. Folic acid: beyond metabolism. *JEBCAM*, 2011 16: 102-113.

Mattson, MP; Shea, TB. Folate and homocysteine metabolism in neural plasticity and neurodegenerative disorders. *Neuroscience,*2003 26, 137-146.

McGrath, J; Brown, A; St Clair, D. Prevention and schizophrenia--the role of dietary factors. *Schizophr. Bull.*, 2011 37(2), 272-283.

Miller, AL. The methylation, neurotransmitter, and antioxidant connections between folate and depression. *Altern. Med. Rev.*, 2008 13(3), 216-226.

Miyamoto, S; LaMantia, AS; Duncan, GE; Sullivan, P; Gilmore, JH; Lieberman, JA. Recent advances in the neurobiology of schizophrenia. *Mol. Interv.*, 2003 3, 27-39.

Molina-Hernández, M; Téllez-Alcántara, NP; Olivera-López, JI; Jaramillo, MT. The folic acid combined with 17-β estradiol produces antidepressant-like actions in ovariectomized rats forced to swim. *Prog. Neuropsychopharmacol. Biol. Psychiatry*, 2011 35(1), 60-66.

Morris, DW; Trivedi, MH; Rush, AJ. Folate and unipolar depression. *J. Altern. Complement. Med.*, 2008 14(3), 277-285.

Muntjewerff, JW; Van der Put, N; Eskes, T; Ellenbroek, B; Steegers, E; Blom, H; Zitman, F. Homocysteine metabolism and B-vitamins in schizophrenic patients: low plasma folate as a possible independent risk factor for schizophrenia. *Psychiatry Res.*, 2003 121(1), 1-9.

Muntjewerff, JW; Hoogendoorn, ML; Kahn, RS; Sinke, RJ; Den Heijer, M; Kluijtmans, LA; Blom, HJ. Hyperhomocysteinemia, methylenetetrahydrofolate reductase 677TT genotype, and the risk for schizophrenia: a Dutch population based case-control study. *Am. J. Med. Genet. B Neuropsychiatr. Genet.*, 2005 135B, 69-72.

Muntjewerff, JW; Kahn, RS; Blom, HJ; den Heijer, M. Homocysteine, methylenetetrahydrofolate reductase and risk of schizophrenia: a meta-analysis. *Mol. Psychiatry*, 2006 11, 143-149.

Nahas, R; Sheikh, O. Complementary and alternative medicine for the treatment of major depressive disorder. *Can. Fam. Physician*, 2011 57(6), 659-663.

Nanri, A; Mizoue, T; Matsushita, Y; Sasaki, S; Ohta, M; Sato, M; Mishima, N. Serum folate and homocysteine and depressive symptoms among Japanese men and women. *Eur. J. Clin. Nutr.*, 2010 64, 289-296.

Osher, Y; Sela, BA; Levine, J; Belmaker, RH. Elevated homocysteine levels in euthymic bipolar disorder patients showing functional deterioration. *Bipolar. Disord.*, 2004 6, 82-86.

Ozbek, Z; Kucukali, CI; Ozkok, E; Orhan, N; Aydin, M; Kilic, G; Sazci, A; Kara, I. Effect of the methylenetetrahydrofolate reductase gene polymorphisms on homocysteine, folate and vitamin B12 in patients with bipolar disorder and relatives. *Prog. Neuropsychopharmacol. Biol. Psychiatry*, 2008 32, 1331-1337.

Papakostas, GI; Petersen, T; Mischoulon, D; Ryan, JL; Nierenberg, AA; Bottiglieri, T; Rosenbaum, JF; Alpert, JE; Fava, M. Serum folate, vitamin B12, and homocysteine in major depressive disorder, Part 1: predictors of clinical response in fluoxetine-resistant depression. *J. Clin. Psychiatry*, 2004a 65(8), 1090-1095.

Papakostas, GI; Petersen, T; Mischoulon, D; Green, CH; Nierenberg, AA; Bottiglieri, T; Rosenbaum, JF; Alpert, JE; Fava, M. Serum folate, vitamin B12, and homocysteine in major depressive disorder, Part 2: predictors of relapse during the continuation phase of pharmacotherapy. *J. Clin. Psychiatry*, 2004b 65(8), 1096-1098.

Papakostas, GI; Petersen, T; Lebowitz, BD; Mischoulon, D; Ryan, JL; Nierenberg, AA; Bottiglieri, T; Alpert, JE; Rosenbaum, JF; Fava, M. The relationship between serum folate, vitamin B12, and homocysteine levels in major depressive disorder and the timing of improvement with fluoxetine. *Int. J. Neuropsychopharmacol.*, 2005 8(4), 523-528.

Passeri, M; Cuciniotta, D; Abate, G; Senin, U; Ventura, A. Oral 5-methyltetrahydrofolic acid in senile organic mental disorders with depression: results of a double-blind multicenter study. *Ageing Clin. Exp. Res.*, 1993 5, 63-71.

Petronijević, ND; Radonjić, NV; Ivković, MD; Marinković, D; Piperski, VD; Duricić, BM; Paunović, VR. Plasma homocysteine levels in young male patients in the exacerbation and remission phase of schizophrenia. *Prog. Neuropsychopharmacol. Biol. Psychiatry*, 2008 32(8), 1921-1926.

Porsolt, RD; Bertin, A; Jalfre, M. Behavioral despair in mice: a primary screening test for antidepressants. *Arch. Int. Pharmacodyn. Ther.*, 1977 229(2), 327-336.

Prince, M; Patel, V; Saxena, S; Maj, M; Maselko, J; Phillipl, MR; Rahman, A. No health without mental health. *Lancet*, 2007 370, 859-877.

Ramaekers, VT; Blau, N. Cerebral folate deficiency. *Dev. Med. Child Neurol.*, 2004 46(12), 843-851.

Resler, G; Lavie, R; Campos, J; Mata, S; Urbina, M; García, A; Apitz, R; Lima, L. Effect of folic acid combined with fluoxetine in patients with major depression on plasma homocysteine and vitamin B12, and serotonin levels in lymphocytes. *Neuroimmunomodulation*, 2008 15(3), 145-152.

Reynolds, EH; Preece, JM; Bailey, J; Coppen, A. Folate deficiency in depressive illness. *Br. J. Psychiatry,* 1970 117(538), 287-292.

Reynolds, E. Vitamin B12, folic acid, and the nervous system. *Lancet Neurol.*, 2006 5(11), 949-960.

Roberts, SH; Bedson, E; Hughes, D; Lloyd, K; Menkes, DB; Moat, S; Pirmohamed, M; Slegg, G; Thome, J; Tranter, R; Whitaker, R; Wilkinson, C; Russell, I. Folate augmentation of treatment - evaluation for depression (FolATED): protocol of a randomised controlled trial. *BMC Psychiatry*, 2007 7, 65.

Roffman, JL; Weiss, AP; Purcell, S; Caffalette, CA; Freudenreich, O; Henderson, DC; Bottiglieri, T; Wong, DH; Halsted, CH; Goff, DC. Contribution of methylenetetrahydrofolate reductase (MTHFR) polymorphisms to negative symptoms in schizophrenia. *Biol. Psychiatry*, 2008 63, 42-48.

Rummel, C; Kissling, W; Leucht, S. Antidepressants as add-on treatment to antipsychotics for people with schizophrenia and pronounced negative symptoms: a systematic review of randomized trials. *Schizophr. Res.*, 2005 80, 85-97.

Saedisomeolia, A; Djalali, M; Moghadam, AM; Ramezankhani, O; Najmi, L. Folate and vitamin B12 status in schizophrenic patients. *JRMS,* 2011 16, 437-441.

Skarupski, KA; Tangney, C; Li, H; Ouyang, B; Evans, DA; Morris, MC. Longitudinal association of vitamin B-6, folate, and vitamin B-12 with depressive symptoms among older adults over time. *Am. J. Clin. Nutr.*, 2010 92(2), 330-335.

Shiah, IS; Yatham, LN. Serotonin in mania and in the mechanism of action of mood stabilizers: a review of clinical studies. *Bipolar. Disord.*, 2000 2, 77-92.

Stahl, SM. Novel therapeutics for depression: L-methylfolate as a trimonoamine modulator and antidepressant-augmenting agent. *CNS Spectr.* 12(10):739-44, 2007.

Steru, L; Chermat, R; Thierry, B; Simon, P. The tail suspension test: a new method for screening antidepressants in mice. *Psychopharmacology (Berl.)*, 1985 85(3), 367-370.

Smith, AM; Picciano, MF; Deering, RH. Folate supplementation during lactation: maternal folate status, human milk folate content, and their relationship to infant folate status. *J. Pediatr. Gastroenterol. Nutr.*, 1983 2, 622- 628.

Smits, LJM; Essed, GM. Short interpregnancy intervals and unfavourable pregnancy outcome: role of folate depletion. *Lancet*, 2001 358, 2074-2077.

Smits, L; Pedersen, C; Mortensen, P; Van Os J. Association between short birth intervals and schizophrenia in the offspring. *Schizophr. Res.*, 2004 70(1), 49-56.

Susser, E; Neugebauer, R; Hoek, HW; Brown, AS; Lin, S; Labovitz, D; Gorman, JM. Schizophrenia after prenatal famine. Further evidence. *Arch. Gen. Psychiatry*, 1996 53(1), 25-31.

Skarupski, KA; Tangney, C; Li, H; Ouyang, B; Evans, DA; Morris, MC. Longitudinal association of vitamin B-6, folate, and vitamin B-12 with depressive symptoms among older adults over time. *Am. J. Clin. Nutr.*, 2010 92(2), 330-335.

Swann, AC. Long-term treatment in bipolar disorder. *J. Clin. Psychiatry*, 2005 66 (1), 7-12.

Tolmunen, T; Voutilainen, S; Hintikka, J; Rissanen, T; Tanskanen, A; Viinamäki, H; Kaplan, GA; Salonen JT. Dietary folate and depressive symptoms are associated in middle-aged Finnish men. *J. Nutr.*, 2003 133(10), 3233-3236.

Walker, JG; Mackinnon, AJ; Batterham, P; Jorm, AF; Hickie, IB; McCarthy, A; Fenech, M; Christensen, H. Mental health literacy, FA and vitamin B12, and physical activity for the prevention of depression in older adults: randomised controlled trial. *Br. J. Psychiatry*, 2010 197(1), 45-54.

Wang, G; Dai, J; Mao, J; Zeng, X; Yang, X; Wang, X. Folic acid reverses hyperresponsiveness of LPS-induced chemokine secretion from monocytes in patients with hyperhomocysteinemia. *Atherosclerosis*, 2005 179, 395-402.

Wesson, VA; Levitt, AJ; Joffe, RT. Change in folate status with antidepressant treatment. *Psychiatry Res.*, 1994 53, 313-322.

Williams, E; Stewart-Knox, B; Bradbury, I; Rowland, I; Pentieva, K; Helander, A; McNulty, H. Effect of folic acid supplementation on mood and serotonin response in healthy males. *Br. J. Nutr.*, 2005 94, 602-608.

Yoshimi, A; Aleksic, B; Kawamura, Y; Takahashi, N; Yamada, S; Usui, H; Saito, S; Ito, Y; Iwata, N; Inada, T; Noda, Y; Yamada, K; Ozaki, N. Gene-wide association study between the methylenetetrahydrofolate reductase gene (MTHFR) and schizophrenia in the Japanese population, with an updated meta-analysis on currently available data. *Schizophr. Res.*, 2010 124, 216-222.

Reviewed by Joana Gil-Mohapel, Ph.D., Division of Medical Sciences, Island Medical Program, University of Victoria, Victoria, BC, Canada.

In: Folic Acid
Editors: Mária Szabó and Eve Varga
ISBN: 978-1-62100-867-5

Chapter III

The Importance of Folic Acid and Its Effects on Fertility, Miscarriage, and Preterm Birth

Jennifer C. Aronica, Monica D. Gorman, Shannon M. Larabee, Jennifer E. Reid and G. Ian Gallicano
Georgetown University School of Medicine,
Georgetown University Medical Center, US

Abstract

Folic acid is an essential micronutrient, and deficiency is linked to an increased risk of neural tube defects in the developing embryo. Knowing the importance of folic acid during embryogenesis, we sought to examine its effects on other aspects of reproduction including fertility, preterm birth, and miscarriage. Studies indicate that folic acid supplementation aids in spermatogenesis. In female reproduction, low homocysteine levels are associated with improved oocyte quality and maturity, as well as increased efficacy of IVF treatments. After evaluating maternal serum folate status and periconceptual folic acid supplementation, researchers found an association between increased folic acid and a reduced risk of preterm birth. However, studies have presented conflicting findings on the role of folic acid in prevention of miscarriage, with some proposing a protective effect of folic acid on the developing fetus. With promising data suggesting that folic acid plays a major role in reproduction outside the realm of neural tube development, more research is needed to clarify the extent of the impact of folic acid supplementation and the mechanism underlying its benefit. Further, supplementation has the potential to reduce healthcare costs associated with these reproductive issues.

Introduction

Folic acid is an essential micronutrient found in green leafy vegetables, legumes, citrus, liver, and kidneys (DeRegil et al., 2011; Lucock, 2000; Obican et al., 2010; Scholl and Johnson, 2000). Key metabolic pathways, such as nucleic acid synthesis and homocysteine remethylation, are dependent upon folate. While folic acid, the synthetic form, and folate, the naturally occurring form, are absorbed as 5-methyltetrahydrofolate (5-methyl-THF) in the gut, intracellularly they are converted to the species dihydrofolate (DHF) or tetrahydrofolate (THF) for use within biochemical pathways (Lucock, 2000).

Folic Acid Biochemistry: During nucleic acid synthesis, the rate-limiting step is the transfer of a methyl unit by thymidine synthase from 5,10-methylenetetrahydrofolate (5,10-methylene-THF), a derivative of folate, to deoxyuridine monophosphate, a precursor to pyrimidine nucleotides. Thymidine synthase levels are high in cells that are in S-phase, and if 5,10-methylene-THF levels are low during the replication of DNA in this phase, synthesis will stop until enough substrate is available (Lucock, 2000; Scholl and Johnson, 2000; Tamura and Picciano, 2006). The remethylation of homocysteine (Hcy) to methionine is dependent on 5,10-methylene-THF much like nucleic acid synthesis. The enzyme 5,10-methylenetetrahydrofolate reductase (5,10-MTHFR) converts 5,10-methylene-THF to 5-methyl-THF, which is then used by methionine synthase in conjunction with vitamin B_{12} to convert Hcy to methionine. Since 5,10-MTHFR is the only enzyme in humans available to make 5-methyl-THF, if either folate or 5,10-methylene-THF is in low quantities, this reaction cannot go forward and Hcy levels will increase (Lucock, 2000; Obican et al., 2010; Scholl and Johnson, 2000; Tamura and Picciano, 2006). These pathways can be found in Figure 1. Folate available for biochemical pathways is shared between two pools, cytosolic and mitochondrial. It fluxes between the two pools, with levels of one affecting the other. Both nucleic acid synthesis and Hcy remethylation draw from the cytosolic pool, thus if there is a general deprivation in one pool, pathways that use folic acid can be disrupted (Lucock, 2000).

Folic Acid, Neural Tube Defects, and Genetic Polymorphisms in Folate Metabolism: Studies have shown that periconceptional folic acid supplementation reduces the risk for neural tube defects (NTDs) (DeRegil et al., 2011; Lucock, 2000; Tamura and Picciano, 2006; Wald et al., 1991), though the exact mechanism for this protective effect is unknown. It is speculated that disruption of DNA synthesis during a time of rapid cellular division due to a lack of folate for precursors can lead to NTDs (Lucock, 2000; Scholl and Johnson, 2000; Siega-Riz et al., 2004). In addition to low environmental folate levels, several genetic polymorphisms (677C → T-MTHFR, 1298A → C-MTHFR) in both heterozygous and homozygous states have been shown to effect normal folate and Hcy metabolism, elevating levels of Hcy and disrupting the availability of 5-methyl-THF for other reactions (Lucock, 2000; Obican et al., 2010; Scholl and Johnson, 2000; Zeisel, 2009). These polymorphisms are associated with a group of NTDs and may play a role in other birth defects and adverse pregnancy outcomes (Lucock, 2000; Scholl and Johnson, 2000).

The Impact of Folic Acid on Pregnancy: A Review: Due to the importance of folic acid in preventing NTDs, fortification of cereals and breads with folic acid has been implemented in some developed countries. Women who are pregnant or planning conception are recommended to take 400 μg to 800 μg of folic acid daily (Lucock, 2000, U.S. Preventive Services Task Force, 2009). Knowing that folate plays essential roles in nucleic acid synthesis and Hcy remeythylation, both key metabolic pathways in developing cells, researchers sought to determine if folic acid may also play a role in other aspects of the developing embryo and pregnancy. Through a review of the literature, we looked at current research on the effects of folic acid on fertility, miscarriage, and preterm birth. Within these three topics, numerous studies have conflicting evidence surrounding the impact of folic acid on pregnancy outcomes.

Folic Acid and Fertility

Impaired fertility affects 10-15% of couples and the severity of impairment is estimated by the length of time that the couple has been unable to conceive (Evers, 2002). Infertility is the complete inability to conceive, while subfertility is the inability of a couple to conceive after one year of unprotected sex during fertile phases of the menstrual cycle. Causes of subfertility include male subfertility, ovulation disturbances, defects in the spermatozoa-cervical mucus interaction, tuboperitoneal disorders, and unexplained subfertility (Evers, 2002).

Male subfertility accounts for 20-26% of subfertility in couples and results from a lack of sperm or abnormal sperm (Evers, 2002). Male subfertility can be diagnosed via semen analysis. A normally fertile male has a sperm count of 20×10^4/mL with at least 50% of the spermatozoa showing progressive motility and 30% exhibiting normal morphology (Evers, 2002). A sperm count below 14.3×10^4, progressive motility less than 28% and normal morphology less than 5% indicate impaired male fertility (Evers, 2002).

Causes of subfertility that originate in females include ovulation disturbances, defects in the cervical mucus, and tuboperitoneal disorders, which account for 18-24%, 9-15% and 11-30% of subfertility respectively. The cause of the remaining 26-30% of subfertility has not yet been identified (Evers, 2002). The two major treatments for impaired fertility are ovarian stimulation and *in vitro* fertilization (IVF). Ovarian stimulation involves use of medications, such as clomiphene, to stimulate multiple eggs to grow in the ovaries, increasing the odds of pregnancy. *In vitro* fertilization involves the combination of sperm and egg outside of the body in a laboratory dish, which is then transferred back into the woman's uterus (2008 ART Report).

A significant number of couples experience problems conceiving and this number is likely to increase since more females are postponing motherhood until later in life. As such, it is important to consider the impact of environmental factors like micronutrient status on fertility. The impact of folate status on subfertility, in particular, has been investigated in numerous studies, although no clear consensus has been reached regarding its efficacy as a treatment option for fertility.

Folic Acid and Male Infertility and Subfertility: Wong et al. (2002) performed a double-blind, randomized controlled trial examining the effects of zinc sulfate and folic acid supplementation on the sperm count of 108 fertile and 103 subfertile men. The median sperm count in the subfertile group increased by 74% after 26 weeks of supplementation while the fertile men showed no significant change in median sperm count (Wong et al., 2002). However, the subfertile men in the groups receiving zinc or folic acid alone did not show a statistically significant increase in sperm count; only the group receiving both supplements in conjunction showed a significantly increased sperm count (Wong et al., 2002). This increase in sperm count suggests that zinc sulfate and folic acid together should improve fertility in subfertile men. In a similar study, Bentivoglio et al. (1993) gave 15 mg folinic acid, a derivative of THF, to 65 infertile men for 3 months and found an increase in the patients' sperm density and motility. Furthermore, of the 65 couples, 24 conceived within 6 months following the treatment, leading to 17 deliveries (Bentivoglio et al., 1993).

A number of authors have investigated the prevalence of a mutation (C677T) in the gene coding for 5,10-MTHFR. This specific mutation reduces the function of the enzyme by 30% in heterozygotes and 70% in homozygotes for the mutation. The three genotypes studied were wild-type (CC), heterozygous (CT), and homozygous (TT) for the mutation. Singh et al. (2004) analyzed DNA from 200 fertile men and 151 infertile men, and found that the allele for the mutation, T, appeared twice as frequently in the infertile population as the fertile population (Singh et al., 2004). Further, there were no homozygotes, TT, in the fertile population while there were six in the infertile population. Thus, they found a statistically significant increase in the frequency of this allele in infertile men and concluded that it is a risk factor for infertility. This genotype results in an altered folate metabolism, increasing the need for folic acid in the diet. In particular, increased folate mitigates the Hcy accumulation in people with this genotype (Singh et al, 2004).

Ebisch et al. (2003) similarly analyzed the prevalence of the T allele in fertile and subfertile men. In contrast to the previous study, they found no statistically significant difference in the presence of the allele in the subfertile population. However, they found that application of zinc sulfate and folate to the wild-type population (CC) of men increased sperm concentration significantly (Ebisch et al., 2003). Singh et al. (2004) conducted their study in India, while Ebisch et al. (2003) completed their research in the Netherlands, where potentially different levels of folate are found in the diet. Studies have indicated that Indian populations have lower levels of folate and higher Hcy levels than Western countries (Singh et al., 2004). Ebsich et al. (2003) did not discuss measuring plasma folate in the fertile and subfertile populations in their methods, suggesting that the initial folate levels of subjects were not characterized. Thus, the European population from the Ebsich et al. (2003) study may have had higher folate levels in their diet prior to the study. Higher folate levels alleviate the effects of the 5,10-MTHFR mutation and could have contributed to the lack of statistically significant differences in fertility between the CT, TT, and CC genotypes in the Ebisch et al. (2003) study. Essentially, men that might have been subfertile with a TT or CT genotype might have been categorized as fertile because their high folate diet compensated for the 5,10-MTHFR mutation.

Furthermore, studies have been conducted in other European populations with similarly conflicting results. Research done by Bezold et al. (2001), which took place in Germany, found a statistically significant difference in the prevalence of the homozygous mutation (TT) in the infertile group (18.8%) versus the fertile group (9.5%). In Italy, Stuppia et al. (2003) found no statistically significant association between the T allele and male infertility as the TT genotype was present in 27.6% of controls and 20.4% of fertile patients. However, in another study in Italy, researchers Paracchini et al. (2006) found the opposite results, that the homozygous TT genotype was associated with infertility. Two additional studies have also been completed in Asia. In Korea, Park et al. (2005) found both a higher frequency of the TT genotype in the infertile population and an association between the TT genotype and azoospermia and severe oligoasthenoteratozoospermia. These results support the theory that dietary differences between Europe and Asia can account for the lack of statistically significant data found by European researchers such as Ebisch et al. (2003) and Stuppia et al. (2003). Researchers Dhillon et al. (2007) in India, on the other hand, found that there was no association between the MTHFR mutation and infertility, but they did measure the plasma folate levels and found that plasma folate levels were lower in infertile men. Also, they found that higher Hcy levels were correlated with infertility. These researchers noted in their discussion that plasma folate levels may be able to modify the effect of the germline MTHFR mutation. Furthermore, they measured plasma folate levels in the participants, but they did not discuss whether the plasma folate levels were significantly higher in participants with the MTHFR mutation who were fertile. The plasma folate levels were recorded as 9.4 ng/mL in the fertile TT homozygotes and 7.6 ng/mL in the infertile TT homozygotes, giving strength to the argument that higher folate levels are mitigating the impact of the mutation. Further, they did note that Hcy levels were significantly higher in the TT homozygotes and suggested Hcy-mediated DNA damage as a potential mechanism for infertility (Dhillon et al., 2007). A summary of these studies is presented in table 1.

Animal studies have affirmed the role of folic acid in spermatogenesis. For example, Mayr et al. (1999) showed that rats deprived of folic acid showed a decreased sperm count. Further, dihydrofolate reducatase inhibitors (Malik et al. 1995) and pyrimethamine (Cosentino et al., 1990, Kalla et al., 1997) reduced sperm count and motility of sperm in mice and prevented pregnancies by these males. In MTHFR knockout mice, researchers found deficiencies in general development, but particularly noted severe oligospermia as well as infertility. However, when they treated these mice with betaine, an alternative methyl donor to 5-methyl-THF, they were able to partially restore spermatogenesis and fertility in the knockout mice (Kelly et al., 2005).

The application of folic acid and zinc sulfate has shown a consistently positive effect on sperm count. Low plasma folate and high homocysteine levels are correlated with infertility. The 5,10-MTHFR mutation that impairs folate metabolism has also been implicated as a risk factor for infertility, again potentially indicating the importance of folate for spermatogenesis. Studies conflict on this point, but more population studies with genomic analysis should be completed that include an initial characterization of plasma folate and Hcy levels to rule out prior nutrition as a confounding factor. With promising data regarding folate supplementation, further study is merited and recommending zinc and folate supplementation to males suffering from impaired fertility seems justified.

Table 1. MTHFR C677T Mutation and Male Fertility

Study	Paper Conclusion
Bezold et al. 2001	Found that the homozygous TT mutation was statistically more prevalent in the infertile population
Ebisch et al. 2003	No statistical significance between fertile and subfertile populations with 677T alleles
Stuppia et al. 2003	No statistical significance between TT mutations and and infertility
Singh et al. 2004	677T mutation twice as common in infertile population and no homozygous TT mutations found in fertile population
Park et al. 2005	Found a higher incidence of TT in the infertile population and noted an association between TT mutations and structural sperm defects
Paracchini et al. 2006	Found that homozygous TT mutation as associated with infertility
Dhillion et al. 2007	No association between 677T mutations and infertility but noted that plasma folate levels were lower and Hcy levels were higher in infertile men

Table 2. MTHFR C677T Mutation and Female Fertility

Study	Conclusion
Ebisch et al. 2006	IVF patients with increased follicular Hcy levels had decreased embryo quality
Thaler et al. 2006	IVF patiets with 677T mutation and older than 35 produced significantly fewer oocytes and required higher hormone doses for ovulation

Folic Acid and Female Subfertility: Little is known about the effects of folic acid on female fertility. Szymanski and Kazdepka-Zieminska (2003) measured Hcy levels in the follicular fluids of patients undergoing IVF treatments and treated half of these subjects with folic acid supplements. They found that elevated levels of Hcy in follicular fluids can be corrected by supplementation. Further, the oocytes that developed in a low Hcy environment showed greater maturity and quality (Szymanski and Kazdepka-Zieminska, 2003). While this increase in oocyte quality and maturity would indicate that folic acid supplementation would help increase fertility, the study did not directly examine whether this reduction in Hcy improved the patients' chances of becoming pregnant.

One study by Thaler et al. (2006) did suggest that folate metabolism has an impact on fertility treatments. Subjects who were homozygous or heterozygous for the 5,10-MTHFR mutation (CT, TT) and older than 35 produced significantly fewer oocytes and required higher hormone doses for ovulation induction in IVF therapy (Thaler et al., 2006). In another IVF study, Ebisch et al. (2006) found that increased follicular Hcy concentration was correlated with decreased embryo quality on day three after IVF. Folic acid supplementation can lower Hcy levels in the follicular fluid and low Hcy levels are associated with improved IVF treatment outcomes. A summary of these studies are presented in table 2.

Thus, while there is an association between folic acid supplementation and improvement in IVF procedures, a direct study with a control population not receiving folic acid would be the most accurate way to determine its impact on IVF treatments. However, studies measuring IVF treatment outcomes cannot ethically deprive folic acid supplementation given its necessity in pregnancy to prevent NTDs.

On the other hand, animal studies using a folic acid deprived control population can be conducted. Folic acid deprivation in monkeys caused degeneration of Graffian follicles, a depletion of granulosa cells and a reduction of the corpus luteum (Mohanty and Das, 1982). Similarly, rats fed a folate-free diet for 16 weeks before mating showed decreased folate concentrations and none were able to conceive (Mooij et al., 1992). Thus, the impact of folate deprivation on fertility reiterates its role in oocyte health and fertility in general.

Folic Acid and its Impact on the Occurrence of Miscarriage

Miscarriage, or spontaneous abortion, is a common adverse pregnancy outcome that affects 15-20% of women who know they are pregnant. However, up to 50% of all eggs that are fertilized are spontaneously aborted before a woman even knows she is pregnant (www.ncbi.nlm.nih.gov). Due to these alarming statistics, much research has been conducted in order to determine specific lifestyle and dietary choices that end in miscarriage. Because of the lack of an appropriate sample population, many causes of miscarriage still remain unknown. Interestingly, folic acid has come to the forefront of this issue and its relation to miscarriage has become quite controversial due to conflicting results in several similar research trials.

Early research surrounding folic acid revolved around the use of the dietary supplement as a protective agent that decreases the risk of NTDs in a developing fetus (Czeizel et al., 1994). The discovery of this preventative use of periconceptional folic acid forced researchers to investigate the other possible adverse pregnancy outcomes that could be affected by folic acid use. In a randomized controlled trial that analyzed pregnancy outcomes of 5,502 females, Czeizel et al. (1994) worked to determine the effects of periconceptional multivitamins, which included 0.8 mg folic acid, versus trace element supplementation. Both types of dietary supplements were administered for at least 28 days prior to conception, intake was continued until the 12th week of gestation, and the participants agreed to discontinue any other vitamin use. The participants were excluded if they exhibited infertility or were pregnant at the start of the study. There was no significant variation in the demographic factors between the two groups that were studied. End results of the pregnancies were obtained from the participants, as well as from the medical facilities where they received their care (Czeizel et al., 1994).

The researchers determined the number of pregnancies, terminations, fetal deaths, and recorded low birth weight and the sex ratio. The fetal deaths were divided into four distinct categories that included chemical pregnancy, ectopic pregnancy, miscarriage, and stillbirth (Table 3). Although there was no significant difference in the rate of the individual categories of fetal death between the two groups, the total rate of fetal death was significantly higher in the multivitamin group. When analyzed individually, the proportion of intrauterine death was 40.2% in the multivitamin group and 38.2% in the trace element group. In addition, there was no significant difference observed in the gestational age of the miscarriage between the two groups, with the maximum gestational age being the 11th-12th week in both groups. Other differences in pregnancy outcomes analyzed were not significant, except the observation of increased fertility with multivitamin use (Czeizel et al., 1994).

Table 3. *Pregnancy outcomes.* Modified from Czeizel et al. (1994). The outcomes of all of the pregnancies analyzed in the multivitamin and trace element groups. Termination refers to selective abortion by choice. Four types of fetal deaths were categorized

Pregnancy Category	Multivitamin (including folic acid)	Trace Elements (no folic acid)
Termination	9	19
Fetal death		
Chemical pregnancy	55	40
Ectopic pregnancy	7	4
Miscarriage	301	251
Stillbirth	11	9
Total Fetal Death	374	304
Live birth	2410	2337
Total	2782	2660

Czeizel et al. (1994) attributed the slight increase in fetal death observed in the multivitamin + folic acid group to chance. However, later analyses served to reinvestigate this idea (Hook and Czeizel, 1997). In addition, the researchers questioned the validity of including chemical pregnancies in the analysis, because they consist of a positive pregnancy test without evidence of an intrauterine pregnancy. Only a few of the chemical pregnancies were proven by ultrasound. Without including the chemical pregnancies in the analysis of fetal death, the difference in the rates was no longer significant (Czeizel et al., 2001).

Other studies, such as the Medical Research Council Vitamin Study, yielded similar findings regarding increased rates of miscarriage with supplemental folic acid use (Wald et al., 1991). This was a randomized, double-blind study conducted to determine whether supplementation with folic acid or a multivitamin at the time of conception could prevent NTDs. The control and sample groups both consisted of women who were at high risk of having a pregnancy with a NTD, due to the fact that they had a prior pregnancy with a NTD. Like other studies on NTDs, the MRC Study found that folic acid prevents the occurrence of the defect. Also, in the reported data there was a relative risk of increase in abortion that was declared by the investigators to not be statistically significant (Wald et al., 1991).

But, in a later investigation by Hook and Czeizel (1997) that compared the Czeizel et al. study (1994) to the MRC study (Wald et al., 1991), a similarity in the rate of occurrence of miscarriage among studied populations was seen. This similarity provides evidence to support the idea that folic acid supplementation may actually increase the rate of the miscarriage. Thus, these studies seem to present somewhat paradoxical suggestions by concluding that folic acid supplements are necessary to decrease the rate of NTDs, however they may increase the chance of a miscarriage. The term terathanasia has been used to describe drugs that may reduce the occurrence of birth defects by spontaneously aborting affected fetuses (Hook and Czeizel, 1997), and folic acid may be one such agent. Therefore, the supposed increase in miscarriage seen with folic acid supplementation may be due to its impact as a protective agent. Instead of being allowed to continue to term, fetuses with birth defects are spontaneously aborted early in development (Hook and Czeizel, 1997).

In 2000, Windham et al. presented a prospective study in which they confirmed the association between miscarriage and multivitamin or folic acid use (Windham et al., 2000). This analysis initiated a wave of debate amongst researchers, who, despite supposed correlation with miscarriage wanted the public to understand the benefits of folic acid use and its very important preventative implications. E.B. Hook (Hook, 2000) first responded to the controversy by introducing the term "pseudoabortifacient." The pseudoabortifacient effect is defined by Hook as the apparent increase in the number of abortions due to the promotion of survival until recognition of not-yet-aborted conceptuses. This means that folic acid allows the pregnancy to continue on a little longer, until when the pregnancy is actually recognized, instead of terminating before the woman even knows she is pregnant. This was proposed in order to defend folic acid against being termed a true abortifacient, although Hook suggests this may be possible, but that more research must be done before public policy concerning the recommended periconceptional supplementation of folic acid is changed (Hook, 2000). Additionally, Hook further supported the idea of folic acid as a pseudoabortifacient through in-depth statistical analysis of previous research (Hook, 2001).

The aforementioned studies also include the use of multivitamins, instead of just folic acid supplements. Many investigators propose that another compound within the multivitamin may be responsible for this supposed effect and that the association between folic acid and miscarriage is unjustified (Wald and Hackshaw, 2001). These researchers dismiss the idea that the relationship is statistically significant and stress the fact that other vitamins included in the supplements may be to blame (Wald and Hackshaw, 2001). Also, A.E. Czeizel further supported the idea that the slight increase in fetal death has no real clinical importance (Czeizel, 2001). Therefore, several researchers have hence set forth to exclusively test the effect of folic acid alone on spontaneous abortion. Gindler et al. (2001) analyzed data collected during a public health campaign done by the Chinese Ministry of Health to prevent NTDs. During the campaign, women were asked to take 400 μg of folic acid and no other vitamins and minerals. The women who took the pills were compared to those participants that did not. Out of the 23,806 pregnant women, 2155 (9.1%) experienced a miscarriage. The rates of miscarriage were similar for those who took a folic acid supplement and those who did not, even after the results were adjusted for differences in age and occupation. Also, the differences in gestational age at miscarriage did not vary significantly between the two groups. Thus, there was no evidence for increased or decreased risk of miscarriage found in this study (Gindler et al., 2001).

In all of the previously mentioned studies, a measurement of plasma folate levels was not included in the research. Therefore, the researchers did not account for the fact that folate levels shift throughout pregnancy (George et al., 2002). In addition, there was a need for karyotype analysis of the spontaneously aborted fetuses in order to determine the cause of miscarriage. In a large, population-based, case-controlled study performed by George et al. (2002), the association between plasma folate levels and spontaneous abortion was analyzed. This study was performed in Sweden, where there was no folic acid fortification of food, so that the true impact of a folate deficiency could be determined. The women self-reported their daily folic acid supplementation, which was defined as 400μg per day. At the time of miscarriage, the plasma folate levels were obtained and intrauterine tissue was sent for karyotype analysis. These participants were compared to control participants, who were matched in gestational age (George et al., 2002).

After controlling for confounding factors, such as maternal age, caffeine consumption and smoking, the results indicated that low folate levels increase the risk of spontaneous abortion, while high levels of folate do not increase risk. In addition, no significant difference in folate levels was found between the normal and abnormal karyotype abortions. This study provides important evidence to support the use of folic acid supplements as a preventative mechanism during early pregnancy, and offers contradictory data that opposes results presented in previous studies (George et al., 2002).

All of the evidence presented surrounding the use of periconceptional folic acid and its impact on the occurrence of miscarriage has been conflicting, and more research must be done in order to determine the biological mechanism behind its influence on early pregnancy. Clinical trials are limited in use due to the ethical risks associated with limiting folic acid use in a pregnant population, when its beneficial nature in preventing NTDs is known. Also, most miscarriages occur before a woman knows she is pregnant, so the protective effect of folic acid could be even larger than expected. Therefore, more research must be conducted in the laboratory to discover the biological role of folic acid in fetal development and whether it serves as a protective agent.

Folic Acid and Preterm Birth

In comparison to infants born at full-term, those born preterm, at a gestation period of 20 weeks, 0 days – 36 weeks, 6 days, are at an increased risk of dying as infants, demonstrating poor growth, and suffering from neurodevelopmental problems (Russell et al., 2007). In addition, immature preterm infants require longer hospitalizations and in 2001 cost the United States an estimated $5.8 billion, accounting for 47% of the costs of infant hospitalizations and 27% of pediatric stays (Russell et al., 2007). More notably, in 2005, the Institute of Medicine estimated the costs associated with preterm delivery to be $26.2 billion, or $51,600 per infant born preterm (Behrman et al., 2006). In 2004, 12.5% of births were defined as a preterm delivery, illustrating the need to investigate ways to decrease the incidence of preterm births (Behrman et al., 2006). Interestingly, early studies, where researchers administered folic acid supplements to pregnant women, found that this supplementation increased the duration of gestation (Baumslag et al., 1970; Blot et al., 1981). In order to develop interventions aimed at preventing preterm deliveries, it is necessary to have an understanding of potential causes of preterm births, one of which may be low maternal folic acid.

Maternal Serum Folate Species in the First and Second Trimesters: Bodnar et al. (2010) examined the relationship between maternal folate status and the risk of preterm birth and spontaneous preterm birth, which they defined as a preterm delivery occurring after preterm labor. After taking blood samples at less than 16 weeks gestation of 313 pregnant women, the researchers measured three markers of folate species in serum, 5-methyl-THF, 5-formyltetrahydrofolate (5-formyl-THF), and folic acid concentration. There were 40 cases of preterm birth in the cohort and after adjusting for race, education, smoking, and obesity, women with the highest total folate concentrations, which were comprised mostly of 5-methyl-THF and 5-formyl-THF, had a 60% reduction in the risk of preterm birth and an 80% reduction in spontaneous preterm birth (Bodnar et al., 2010). In addition, Scholl et al. (1996) found that at 28 weeks gestation, women with a low serum folate were at an increased risk for preterm delivery and delivering a low birth weight infant. These findings were also confirmed when Siega-Riz et al. (2004) found that women in their second trimester, between 24-29 weeks gestation, with a total folate serum concentration below 16.3 ng/mL and intake of dietary folate less than 500 μg/day had a 50-90% increase in preterm and spontaneous preterm birth. The findings of these studies also show the need to develop a biological mechanism for how a folate deficiency could lead to preterm birth and whether the level of different types of folate species in the serum, such as 5-methyl-THF and 5-formyl-THF, are involved (Bodnar et al., 2010). Bodnar et al. (2010), Scholl et al. (1996), and Siega-Riz et al. (2004) found that low maternal serum folate status was associated with increased risk of preterm birth. However, these were observational studies that could not exclude all confounders, such as physical activity, family support, and education that can be accounted for in randomized controlled trials.

Maternal Serum Homocysteine Levels: Studies have also explored the relationship between Hcy levels and preterm births as a result of preterm premature rupture of amniotic membranes, PPROM (Knudtson et al., 2004; Kramer et al., 2009). It is thought that PPROM is caused in part by collagen abnormalities and elevated Hcy levels which have been associated with abnormal collagen cross-linking, leading researchers to hypothesize that elevated Hcy is related to PPROM (Ferguson et al., 2001; Knudtson et al. 2004). In addition, mothers who give birth to preterm infants have been shown to be at an increased risk of dying from coronary heart disease, suggesting that vasculopathic risk factors may underlie preterm birth (Kramer et al., 2009). Knudtson et al. (2004) tested the hypothesis that serum Hcy levels, a marker of cardiovascular health, would be higher in women with PPROM when compared to a control group. The researchers examined 99 cases of PPROM from two different prospective cohort studies with gestational ages between 24 – 32 weeks and found that serum Hcy levels did not differ significantly between those with PPROM deliveries and a comparison group (Knudtson et al., 2004). Moreover, Gomes et al. (2010) found that concentrations of total homocysteine (tHcy) in small-for-gestational age (SGA) preterm neonates and appropriate-for-gestation (AGA) preterm neonates, as measured from venous umbilical cord plasma, did not differ significantly among the groups. Their findings suggest that tHcy does not play a role in the intrauterine growth retardation that can be seen in preterm infants (Gomes et al., 2010).

Conversely, a recent study examining whether women who give birth to preterm infants are more likely to die from heart attack or stroke also looked at the relationship between elevated Hcy levels and preterm birth (Kramer et al., 2009). After examining 207 spontaneous preterm births in comparison to 441 controls, the researchers found a significant difference between Hcy levels in preterm birth mothers compared to controls, 4.0 μmol/L and 3.7 μmol/L respectively. Their results suggest that elevated Hcy levels could be a marker for placental vascular changes leading to PPROM or preterm labor (Kramer et al., 2009). Interestingly, the researchers noted they did not find a statistically significant relationship between plasma folate levels and preterm birth despite the fact that the women with low folate levels did have higher Hcy levels (Kramer et al., 2009). An explanation for this finding is that the cohort was from Canada where fortification of flour was mandated and the majority of the women in the study were taking folic acid and/or multivitamins. Therefore, at the time of blood sampling, their supplement use may have prevented the researchers from observing a significant association between plasma folate and preterm birth that may be present in unsupplemented women (Kramer et al., 2009).

While Knudtson et al. (2004) did not find a significant difference between Hcy levels in women who delivered preterm, they used a small population of only 99 cases. Had they used a larger study population they may have reached statistical significance. On the other hand, the larger Kramer et al. (2009) study did find a significant difference between Hcy levels. These conflicting findings demonstrate the need for larger study populations and research on the mechanism of folate during pregnancy in relation to Hcy levels that could lead to an increased incidence of PPROM. A summary of folate and Hcy status in relation to risk of preterm birth can be found in table 4.

Folic Acid Supplementation in Preconception and Late Pregnancy: Not only have studies found a relationship between maternal folate status and preterm birth, as described previously, but results also suggest an association between folic acid supplementation before and during pregnancy with a decreased risk of preterm delivery (Bukowski et al., 2009; Czeizel et al., 2010; Johnson et al. 2005). More recently, in a study population of 34,480 women who were previously enrolled in a prospective cohort study, researchers investigated whether folic acid supplementation before pregnancy reduced the risk of preterm birth (Bukowski et al., 2009).

Within their first three months of pregnancy, participants reported if they took folic acid supplements prior to conception and the duration of supplementation (Bukowski et al., 2009). A spontaneous preterm birth was defined in this study as a preterm birth not associated with complications that necessitated an early delivery, such as preeclampsia or chromosomal abnormalities (Bukowski et al., 2009).

Table 4. Serum folate and serum Hcy levels and their relation to risk of preterm birth

Study	Paper Conclusion
Serum Folate Levels	
Scholl et al. 1996	Found that low serum folate in the second trimester had an increase in risk for preterm delivery and low birth weight
Seiga-Riz et al. 2004	Found that low serum folate in the second trimester increased the risk of preterm and spontaneous preterm birth
Kramer et al. 2009	Did not find a relation between serum folate levels and preterm birth
Bondar et al. 2010	When measuring serum in the first and second trimester, higher early serum folate correlated with a lower risk for preterm birth, serum
Serum Hcy Levels	
Knudtson et al. 2004	During the second and third trimesters, there was no correlation between serum Hcy levels and PPROM and/or preterm birth
Kramer et al. 2009	Found that mothers who had preterm births also had higher serum Hcy levels
Gomes et al. 2010	Total Hcy levels from umbilical cord blood in neonates did not differ between small-for-gestational and appropriate-for-gestational age preterm neonates

Of the participants, 1,658 had spontaneous preterm deliveries before 37 weeks and 160 before 32 weeks. After analyses, results showed that the risk of spontaneous preterm delivery between 20-28 weeks was reduced by 70% in women who had taken folic acid supplements for more than a year compared to women who had not reported supplement use (Bukowski et al., 2009). Also, long-term supplementation reduced the risk of preterm delivery between 28-32 weeks by 50% (Bukowski et al., 2009). Despite these findings, the researchers noted that folic acid supplementation did not decrease the risk of preterm delivery after 32 weeks and supplementation for less than one year did not reduce the risk of preterm birth (Bukowski et al., 2009).

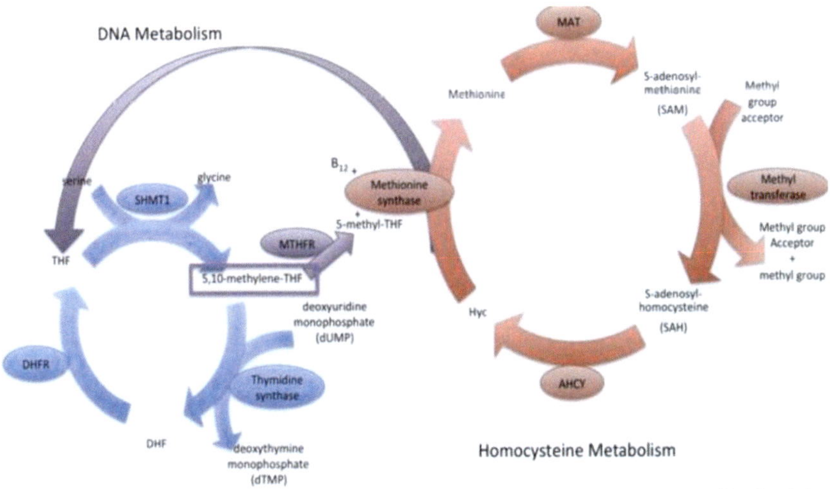

Abbreviations: AHCY – *S*-adenosylhomocysteine hydrolase; DHF – dihydrofolate; DHFR – dihydrofolate reductase; Hyc – homocysteine; MAT – methionine adenosyltransferase; MTHFR – methylenetetrahydrofolate reductase; THF – tetrahydrofolate.

Figure 1. *Relevant folate-dependent one-carbon metabolism.* The use of folic acid as discussed in the introduction in the DNA and homocysteine metabolism cycles is shown here. The common precursor 5,10-methylene-THF is highlighted to show its importance in both pathways. Purine metabolism and other pathways not discussed are not included in this figure.

In contrast, a study conducted in Hungary found results suggesting that continued folic acid supplementation throughout the third trimester significantly reduced the rate of preterm births (Czeizel et al., 2010). The study looked at 38,151 newborns and examined how maternal intake of folic acid alone or in conjunction with multivitamins affected preterm birth when compared to a reference group that did not take any supplements (Czeizel et al., 2010). The researchers found that in the folic acid only group, there was a significant decrease in the rate of preterm births (7.6%) when compared to the reference group (11.8%). Moreover, their results showed that folic acid supplementation alone during the third trimester resulted in a significant reduction in the rate of preterm births to 4.8% (Czeizel et al., 2010).

In addition, Johnson et al. (2005) investigated whether a deletion polymorphism in the dihydrofolate reductase (DHFR) gene can increase the risk of preterm birth. DHFR is needed in a mechanism used by cells to convert the folic acid found in supplements into a usable derivative involved in DNA synthesis. The researchers also looked at the association between folic acid intake and this DHFR polymorphism gene deletion. Not only did they find that pregnant women with this deletion allele had a significantly greater risk for preterm birth, but women with the deletion allele and a folic acid intake of < 400μg/day had an increased risk for preterm delivery and delivering a low birth weight infant than women without the allele and a folic acid intake > 400μg/ day (Johnson et al., 2005).

These studies found an association between low folic acid supplementation and an increased risk of preterm birth, which lends more weight to the fact that supplementation may reduce the risk of preterm birth (Bukowski et al., 2009; Czeizel et al., 2010; Johnson et al., 2005). In addition, their findings illustrate the need to explain the role of folic acid in fetal development and the stages of pregnancy to understand the differing effects of short-term and long-term supplementation on preterm birth.

Conclusion

The current research concerning folic acid and its effect on pregnancy is diverse in its opinions concerning fertility, miscarriage, and preterm birth. Research on miscarriage presents the possibility that folic acid supplementation may increase rates of spontaneous abortion, posing a hazard to the developing embryo (Wald et al., 1991; Czeizel et al., 1994; Windham et al., 2000). However, later studies have shown that there is no effect of folic acid on spontaneous abortions (George et al. 2002), leaving the protective effect of folic acid unclear beyond preventing NTDs (Hook and Czeizel, 1997). More studies that use populations of women who do not take folic acid are needed to determine the role of folic acid in miscarriages, though this study proposal has ethical concerns as folic acid supplementation is recommended to prevent NTDs. In addition, measuring the rate of miscarriage presents a challenge, as most miscarriages occur before a woman realizes she is pregnant. Therefore, continued research must be done in order to find a biological mechanism that is responsible for the effect of folic acid on the developing fetus, especially to perhaps determine its action very early in pregnancy in selecting viable fetuses.

In male subfertility, there is evidence that folic acid supplementation, in combination with zinc, increases sperm count (Wong et al., 2002). Furthermore, folinic acid supplementation has increased patient sperm density and motility as well as the ability to conceive in infertile couples (Bentivoglio et al. 1993). Mutations in 5,10-MTHFR result in impaired folate metabolism and have been associated with subfertility. There is conflict over whether subfertility due to the mutation may be masked if there is high folic acid supplementation in the diet (Singh et al., 2004). Studies investigating the effect of folic acid on female fertility have indicated that low Hcy levels improve oocyte quality and maturity and correlate with increased embryo quality after IVF procedures (Ebisch et al., 2006; Szymanski et al., 2003). Further, subjects with the CC genotype associated with lower Hcy levels needed lower hormone doses for IVF procedures and produced more oocytes (Thaler et al., 2006).

The cost of IVF to both the family and insurance company for a woman under the age of 35 undergoing one cycle of IVF and implanting one embryo costs $24,216 and transferring five embryos costs $41,907. The cost increases for women over 40 (Little et al., 2006). As low Hcy in follicular fluid appears to improve oocyte health and the effectiveness of IVF treatments, ensuring folic acid supplementation could reduce the need to harvest more eggs and implant numerous embryos, ultimately lowering the cost of IVF treatments or reducing their need for in populations where low folate status is the main barrier to pregnancy.

Folic acid supplementation appears to decrease the incidence of preterm birth (Bukowski et al., 2009; Czeizel et al., 2010; Johnson et al., 2005), though the mechanism is poorly understood. Further, high Hcy levels may not only be a marker of low folate status, but also may play an active role in preterm birth (Kramer et al., 2009). There is need for more research to determine if folic acid supplementation quantities need to be varied during pregnancy. Studies looking at folic acid supplementation may be limited due to the ethical concerns of withholding supplementation as a control, though measuring folate or Hcy serum status may be suitable markers for determining total folic acid intake. These studies are necessary as a single preterm infant hospitalization can cost the family and health care system between $15,600 and $65,600 (Russell et al., 2007). Folic acid may potentially be a simple and inexpensive method to reduce the expenses associated with preterm births.

Overall, folic acid supplementation could be a cost effective method to reduce the incidence of subfertility and preterm birth in addition to its known prevention of NTDs. While the role of folic acid in miscarriages is less understood, evidence does not indicate that the current recommendation for folic acid supplementation should be called into question. The current recommendation for folic acid supplementation should be emphasized as it may reduce health care costs surrounding pregnancy.

References

Baumslag, N., Edelsteine, T. and Metz, J. (1970). Reduction of incidence of prematurity by folic acid supplementation in pregnancy. *British Medical Journal, 1,* 16-17.

Behrman, R.E. and Stith Butler, A. editors. (2006). *Institute of Medicine, Committee on Understanding Preterm Birth and Assuring Healthy Outcomes Board on Health Sciences Policy: Preterm Birth—Causes, Consequences, and Prevention.* Washington, DC: National Academies Press.

Bentivoglio, G, Melica, F. and Cristoforoni, P. (1993). Folinic acid in the treatment of human male infertility. *Fertility and Sterility, 60,* 698-701.

Bezold, G., Lange, M. and Peter, R.U. (2001). Homozygous methylenetetrahydrofolate reductase C677T mutation and male infertility. *New England Journal of Medicine, 344,* 1172-3.

Blot, I., Papiernik, E., Kaltwasser, J.P., Werner, E. and Tchernia, G. (1981). Influence of routine administration of folic acid and iron during pregnancy. *Gynecological and Obstetric Investigation, 12,* 294-304.

Bodnar, L.M., Himes, K.P., Venkataramanan, R., Chen, J.Y., Evans, R.W., Meyer, J.L. et al. (2010). Maternal serum folate species in early pregnancy and risk of preterm birth. *American Journal of Clinical Nutrition, 92,* 864-71.

Bukowski, R., Malone, F.D., Porter, F.T., Nyberg, D.A., Comstock, C.H., Hankins, G.D. et al. (2009). Preconceptional folate supplementation and the risk of spontaneous preterm birth: a cohort study. *PLoS Med.* 6, e1000061.

Centers for Disease Control and Prevention, American Society for Reproductive Medicine, Society for Assisted Reproductive Technology. (2010). 2008 Assisted Reproductive Technology Success Rates: National

Summary and Fertility Clinic Reports. Atlanta: U.S. Department of Health and Human Services.

Cosentino, M.J., Pakyz, R.E. and Fried, J. (1990). Pyrimethamine: an approach to the development of a male contraceptive. *Proceedings of the National Academy of Sciences, 87,* 1431-5.

Czeizel, A.E. (2001). Miscarriage and use of multivitamins or folic acid. *American Journal of Medical Genetics, 104,* 179-80.

Czeizel, A.E., Metneki, J. and Dudas, I. (1994). Pregnancy outcomes in a randomized controlled trial of periconceptional multivitamin supplementation. Final report. *Archives of Gynecology and Obstetrics, 255,* 131-139.

Czeizel, A.E., Puho, E.H., Langmar, Z., Acs, N. and Banhidy, F. (2010). Possible association of folic acid supplementation during pregnancy with reduction of preterm birth: a population-based study. *European Journal of Obstetrics and Gynecology and Reproductive Biology, 148,* 135-140.

DeRegil, M.L., Fernandez-Gaxiola, A.C., Dowswell, T. and Pena-Rosas, P.J. (2011). Effects and safety of periconceptional folate supplementation for preventing birth defects. *Cochrane Database of Systematic Reviews. 10.*

Ebisch, I.M., van Heerde, W.L., Thomas, C.M., van der Put, N., Wong, W.Y. and Steegers-Theunissen, R.P. (2003). C677T methylenetetrahydrofolate reductase polymorphism interferes with the effects of folic acid and zinc sulfate on sperm concentration. *Fertility and Sterility, 80,* 1190-1194.

Ebisch, I.M., Peters, W.H., Thomas, C.M., Wetzels, A.M., Peer, P.G. and Steegers-Theunissen, R.P. (2006). Homocysteine, glutathione and related thiols affect fertility parameters in the (sub)fertile couple. *Human Reproduction, 21,* 1725-1733.

Evers, J.L. (2002). Female subfertility. *The Lancet, 360,* 151-159.

Ferguson, S.E., Smith, G.N. and Walker, M.C. (2001). Maternal plasma homocysteine levels in women with preterm premature rupture of membranes. *Medical Hypotheses 56,* 85-90.

George,L., Mills, J.L., Johansson, A.L., Nordmark, A., Olander, B., Granath, F. et al. (2002). Plasma folate levels and risk of spontaneous abortion. *Journal of the American Medical Association, 288,* 1867-1873.

Gindler, J., Li, Z., Berry, R.J., Zheng, J., Correa, A., Sun, X. et al. (2001). Folic acid supplements during pregnancy and risk of miscarriage. *The Lancet, 358,* 796-800.

Gomes, T.S., Lindner, U., Tennekoon, K.H., Karandagoda, W., Gortner, L. and Obeid, R. (2010). Homocystine in small-for-gestational age and appropriate-for-gestational age preterm neonates from mothers receiving folic acid supplementation. *Clinical Chemistry and Laboratory Medicine, 48,* 1157-1161.

Hook, E.B. (2000). Folic acid: abortifacient or pseudoabotifacient? *American Journal of Medical Genetics, 92,* 301-302.

Hook, E.B. (2001). Statistical and logical considerations in evaluating the association of prenatal folic-acid supplementation with pregnancy loss. *American Journal of Medical Genetics, 104,* 181-2.

Hook, E.B. and Czeizel, A.E. (1997). Can terathanasia explain the protective effect of folic acid supplementation on birth defects? *The Lancet, 350,* 513-515.

Johnson, W.G., Scholl, T.O, Spychala, J.R., Buyske, S., Stenroos, E.S. and Chen, X. (2005). Common dihydrofolate reductase 19-base pair deletion allele: a novel risk factor for preterm delivery. *American Journal of Clinical Nutrition, 81,* 664-8.

Kalla, N.R, Saggar, S.K., Puri R. and Metha, U. (1997). Regulation of male fertility by pyrimethamine in adult mice. *Research in Experimental Medicine, 197,* 45-52.

Kelly, T.L.J., Neaga, O.R., Schwahn, Rozen, R. and Trasler, J.M. (2005). Infertility in 5,10-methylenetetrahydrofolate reductase (MTHFR) – deficient male mice is partially alleviated by lifetime dietary betaine supplementation. *Biology of Reproduction, 72*, 667-7.

Knudtson, E.J., Smith, K., Mercer, B.M., Miodovnik, M., Thurnau, G.R., Goldenberg, R.L. et al. (2004). Serum homocysteine levels after preterm premature rupture of the membranes. *American Journal of Obstetrics and Gynecology, 191,* 537-41.

Kramer, M.S., Kahn, S.R., Rozen, R., Evans, R., Platt, R.W., Chen, M.F. et al. (2009). Vasculopathic and thrombophilic risk factors for spontaneous preterm birth. *International Journal of Epidemiology, 38,* 715-723.

Little, S.E., Ratcliffe, J. and Caughey, A.B. (2006). Cost of transferring one through five embryos per *in vitro* fertilization cycle from various payor perspectives. *Obstetrics and Gynecology, 108,* 593-601.

Lucock, M. (2000). Folic acid: nutritional biochemistry, molecular biology, and role in disease processes. *Molecular Genetics and Metabolism, 71,* 121-138.

Malik, N.S., Matlin, S.A., Fried, J., Pakyz and Consentino, M.J. (1995). The contraceptive effects of etoprine on male mice and rats. *Journal of Andrology, 16, 169-74.*

Mayr, C.A., Ingersoll, R., Wallock, L.M. and Ames, B. (1999). Folate levels and the effects of folate deficiency in the reproductive organs of male rats. *The FASEB Journal, 13,* A229.

Mohanty, D., and Das, K.C. (1982). Effect of folate deficiency on the reproductive organs of female rhesus monkeys: a cytomorphological and cytokinetic study. *Journal of Nutrition, 112,* 1565-76.

Mooij, P.N., Wouters, M.G., Thomas, C.M., Doesburg, W.H. and Eskes, T.K.A.B. (1992). Disturbed reproductive performance in extreme folic acid deficient golden hamsters. *European Journal of Obstetrics and Gynecology and Reproductive Biology, 43,* 71-5.

Obican, S.G., Finnell, R.H., Mills, J.L., Shaw, G.M. and Scialli, A.R. (2010). Folic acid in early pregnancy: a public health success story. *The FASEB Journal. 24,* 4167-74.

Paracchini, V., Garte, S. and Taioli, E. (2006). MTHFR C677T polymorphism, GSTM1 deletion and male infertility: a possible suggestion of a gene-gene interaction? *Biomarkers, 11,* 53-60.

Park, J.H., Lee, H.C., Jeong, Y.M., Chung,T.G., Kim, H.J., Kim, N.K. et al.(2005). MTHFR C677T polymorphism associates with unexplained infertile male factors. *Journal of Assisted Reproduction and Genetics, 22,* 361-8.

Russell, R.B., Green, N.S., Steiner, C.A., Meikle, S., Howse, J.L., Poschman, K. et al. (2007). Cost of hospitalization for preterm and low birth weight infants in the United States. *Pediatrics*, *120*, e1-e9.

Scholl, T.O, Hediger, M.L., Scall, J.I., Khoo, C.S. and Fischer, R.L. (1996). Dietary and serum folate: their influence on the outcome of pregnancy. *American Journal of Clinical Nutrition, 63,* 520-525.

Scholl, T.O., and Johnson, W.G. (2000). Folic acid: influence on the outcome of pregnancy. *American Journal of Clinical Nutrition, 71*, 1295S-303S.

Siega-Riz A.M., Savitz, D.A., Zeisel, S.H., Thorp, J.M. and Herring, A. (2004). Second trimester folate status and preterm birth. *American Journal of Obstetrics and Gynecology, 191,* 1851-7.

Singh, K., Singh, S.K., Sah, R., Singh, I. and Raman, R. (2005). Mutation C677T in the methylenetetrahydrofolate reductase gene is associated with male infertility in an Indian population. *International Journal of Andrology, 28,* 115-9.

Stuppia, L., Gatta, V., Scarciolla, O., Colosimo, A., Guanciali-Franchi, P., Calabrese, G. et al. (2003). The methylenetethrahydrofolate reductase (MTHFR) C677T polymorphism and male infertility in Italy. *Journal of Endocrinological Investigation, 26,* 620-2.

Szymanski, W., and Kazdepka-Zieminska, A. (2003). [Effect of homocysteine concentration in follicular fluid on a degree of oocyte maturity]. *Ginekologia Polska, 74,* 1392-6.

Tamura, T., and Picciano, M.F. (2006). Folate and human reproduction. *American Journal of Clinical Nutrition, 83*, 993-1016.

Thaler, C.J., Budiman, H., Ruebsamen, H., Nagel, D. and Lohse, P. (2006). Effects of the common 677C>T mutation of the 5,10-methylenetetrahydrofolate reductase (MTHFR) gene on ovarian responsiveness to recombinant follicle-stimulating hormone. *American Journal of Reproductive Immunology, 55,* 251-8.

U.S. Preventive Services Task Force. (2009). Folic acid for the prevention of neural tube defects: U.S. Preventive Services Task Force recommendation statement. *Annals of Internal Medicine, 150,* 626-31.

Vorvick, L.J., Storck, S. and Zieve, D. editors. Miscarriage [Internet]. Bethesda: National Center for Biotechnology Information [updated 2010 November 21, cited 2011 May 20]. Available from: http://www.ncbi.nlm.nih.gov/pubmedhealth/PMH0002458/.

Wald, N., (1991). Prevention of neural tube defects: results of the Medical Research Council Vitamin Study. MRC Vitamin Study Research Group. *The Lancet, 338,* 131-7.

Wald, N.J., Hackshaw, A.K. (2001). Folic acid and miscarriage: an unjustified risk. *American Journal of Medical Genetics, 98,* 204.

Windham, G.C., Shaw, G.M., Todoroff, K. and Swan, S.H. (2000). Miscarriage and the use of multi-vitamins or folic acid. *American Journal of Medical Genetics, 90,* 260-2.

Wong, W.Y., Merkus, H.M., Thomas, C.M., Menkveld, R., Zielhuis, G.A. and Steegers-Theunissen, R.P. (2002). Effects of folic acid and zinc sulfate on male factor subfertility: a double-blind, randomized, placebo controlled trial. *Fertility and Sterility, 77,* 491-8.

Zeisel, S.H. (2009). Importance of methyl donors during reproduction. *American Journal of Clinical Nutrition 89,* 673S-7S.

In: Folic Acid
Editors: Mária Szabó and Eve Varga

ISBN: 978-1-62100-867-5

Chapter IV

The Actions of Folic Acid in the Prevention of Neural Tube Defects: A Limited Role in Diabetes Mellitus and Epilepsy

Kevin Emmerich[1], Justin King[1], Jacqueline Pham[1], Sunmi Yang[1] and G. Ian Gallicano[1,2]

[1]Georgetown University School of Medicine
[2]Department of Biochemistry and Molecular and Cellular Biology
Georgetown University Medical Center, Washington, DC, US

Abstract

The relationship between folic acid (FA) and neural tube defects (NTDs) has been well documented in the last twenty years. Increased FA intake due to fortification methods have been shown to reduce the incidence of NTDs significantly. While FA's role as a methylating agent has been established, the processes behind the development of NTDs are still being studied. Several proposed mechanisms involving metabolic deficiencies of factors of the remethylation cycle have demonstrated exaggerated behaviors in diseased states. Diabetes mellitus contributes to a higher incidence of NTDs, which can be ameliorated by FA supplementation. Hyperglycemia appears to adversely affect proliferation and normal apoptosis of neural progenitor cells, as well as placental uptake of FA, through mechanisms of oxidative stress. Similar attenuation is seen in the treatment of women with epilepsy. The interaction of FA and antiepileptic drugs (AEDs) presents a complication in the care of pregnancy. AEDs are associated with increased rates of NTDs, thus making prenatal planning imperative. This includes periconceptual FA fortification, administration of the lowest possible dose of AEDs, and antenatal screening for NTDs. Current research supports increased intake of FA in women, especially those in a diseased state. Further research is necessary in order to ascertain the true limits of FA action.

Introduction

Neural tube defects (NTDs) resulting from improper closure of the neural tube within the first month of the development of an embryo are a cause of debilitating and often lethal birth defects. Approximately 4,000 pregnancies and 2,500 live births in the United States each year are affected by spina bifida or anencephaly, the two most common NTDs (Williams *et al.*, 2002). While the underlying mechanisms and risk factors remain in question, studies have shown up to a 72% decrease in the rate of NTD occurrence with periconceptual folic acid (FA) supplementation (Oddy *et al.,* 2007). Statistics such as this have led a number of countries including the United States to mandate the fortification of grains with FA. However, fortification alone has not completely eliminated the occurrence of NTDs. This indicates that rather than a simple deficiency in FA, additional underlying metabolic conditions may contribute to the prevalence of NTDs. In order to better understand the role that FA plays in the development of the neural tube, a great amount of research has been devoted to this field. In an effort to expand on the current understanding of this topic, we will examine the impact that FA has on the prevention of NTDs, the possible mechanisms involved in this process, and areas of research that have exhibited a limited response to FA supplementation.

Epidemiological Studies of Folic Acid Fortification

Due to a better understanding of FA's preventative effects on NTDs, a number of countries began campaigning for FA fortification of grain products in the late twentieth country. By 1992 the United States Public Health Service (USPHS) had made a formal recommendation that women of child bearing age should consume no less than 400 μg of FA per day. Soon after, the Food and Drug Administration (FDA) mandated that all grain products be fortified with 140 μg of FA per 100 g of grain. Following a two-year period of optional compliance, the law went into effect on January 1, 1998. This law provided the basis of a study done by Williams *et al.* to determine the effects of fortification on prevention of the two most common NTDs: spina bifida and anencephaly. Comparing the prevalence of these two neural tube defects in pre- and post-fortification eras proved reassuring for the FDA. The rate of spina bifida and anencephaly decreased 31% and 16%, respectively, from 1995-1996 to 1998-1999 (Williams *et al.*, 2002). This result coincided with Daly's 1997 results comparing maternal red blood cell FA levels and NTD prevalence. FA levels below 150 μg/L in the mother during pregnancy produced NTDs in 6.6 of 1000 live births. Subjects whose FA level matched the USPHS recommendation of 400 μg/L fared markedly better with defects in only 0.8 per 1000 (Daly *et al.*, 1997).

In November of 1998, Canada began its own mandatory fortification only ten months after the United States. Prior to compiling data it was known that a geographical gradient existed in the prevalence of spina bifida. In the eastern, central, and western regions, spina bifida presented in 1.68, 0.98, and 0.53 cases per 1000 live births, respectively. Also the percentage of upper defects in spina bifida cases was higher in the east than west (45.3% to 24.1%). These data implied that there was both a lack of knowledge of FA's preventative effects and lack of resources in the eastern region of Canada. After mandatory fortification, the results from a study conducted by De Wals indicated a 46% decline in all neural tube defects compared to pre-fortification years. These results did not segregate Canada into different regions, due to the fact that the geographical gradient was nearly erased after nationwide fortification. A trend in lesion location also arose in cases of spina bifida. The percentage of upper spinal defects decreased from 32% to 13%. Both the elimination of the regional gradient of all neural tube defects and the decrease in upper spinal spina bifida defects demonstrated that FA fortification was beneficial (De Wals *et al.*, 2008).

Although data about the positive effects of FA in preventing NTDs were becoming available, some countries were more reluctant to make fortification a law. China is responsible for approximately 18,000 of the world's babies born with NTDs each year. The government has yet to mandate fortification at this time but is performing test trials in certain parts of the country. Interestingly, the Chinese are examining rice as the crop of choice to become fortified (De Steur *et al.*, 2010).

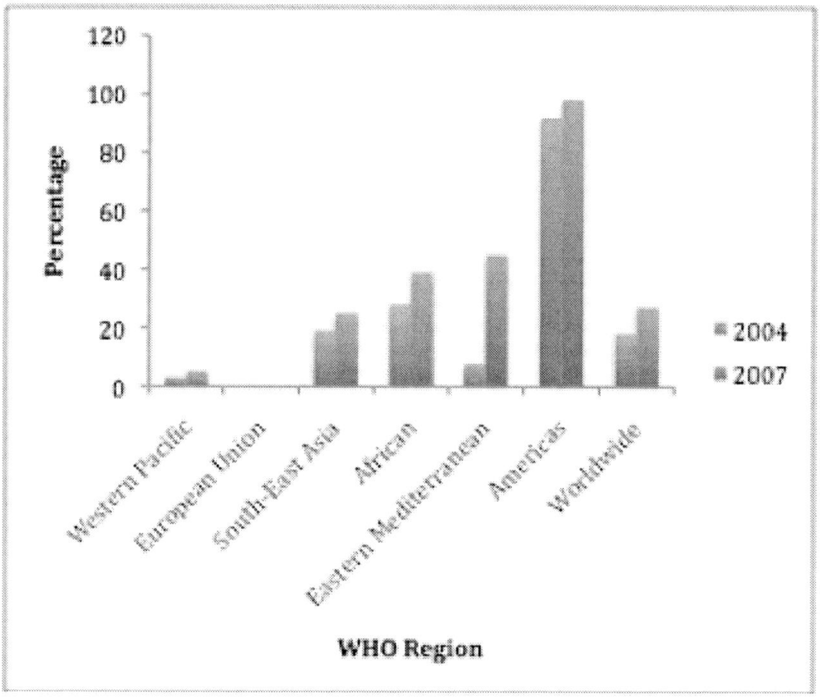

Figure 1. Percentage of wheat flour processed in roller mills that was fortified – worldwide and by World Health Organization (WHO) region, 2004 and 2007 (Centers for Disease Control and Prevention.

Australia implemented voluntary fortification in 1995 (Oddy *et al.*, 2007) but was hesitant to follow what would soon become a North American trend to require it by law (Centers for Disease Control and Prevention). Even with voluntary fortification the reduction of NTDs became significant. Before 1995, the prevalence of NTDs (including both live births and terminations) was 2 cases for every 1000 pregnancies. Just one year into voluntary fortification this number decreased by 30% to 1.4 per 1000. By 1999 over 100 foods had reportedly been fortified including breakfast cereals, fruit juice, and milk. In 2007 the Australian government approved mandatory fortification, which became effective in 2009 (Oddy *et al.*, 2007).

Of all world regions, North and South Americas have shown the most diligence in making FA fortification mandatory in wheat flour products. By 2007, 97% of their countries had done so, as shown by Figure 1.

In contrast, Europe has resisted the FA movement. No country in the European Union has made FA fortification mandatory (Centers for Disease Control and Prevention). Great Britain, among other countries, is concerned for other health risks that arise when the FA dose approaches the milligram level. These include the increased risk for colorectal cancer and the masking of vitamin B12 deficiencies (Food Standards Agency). Overall, it is estimated that FA fortification has reduced the worldwide prevalence of NTDs by 46% (Običan *et al.*, 2010). Table 1 includes the prevalence of NTDs for a number of countries before and after making fortification mandatory.

Table 1. Prevalence of neural tube defects before and after mandatory fortification in the United States (Williams, *et al.*, 2002), Canada (De Wals, *et al.*, 2008), Costa Rica (Chen and Rivera, 2004), Jordan (Amarin and Obeidat, 2010), Chile (Hertrampf and Cortés, 2004), Brazil and Argentina (López-Camela, *et al.*, 2009), Australia (Oddy, *et al.*, 2006), and South Africa (Sayed, *et al.*, 2008)

	Mandatory Fortification	NTD Prevalence Pre-Fortification per 1000 births	NTD Prevalence Post-Fortification per 1000 births	Improvement
United States	1998	0.76	0.56	26%
Canada	1998	0.86	0.40	36%
Costa Rica	1997/1999**	9.70	6.30	35%
Jordan	2002	1.85	0.95	49%
Chile	2000	1.70	1.00	40%
Brazil	2004	3.14	2.43	23%
Argentina	2003	2.45	1.23	50%
Australia*	N/A	2.00	1.40	30%
South Africa	2003	1.41	0.98	31%

*At time of study, Australia had only implemented voluntary fortification

**Puerto Rico mandated fortification of wheat flour in 1997 and corn flour in 1999

Physiological Mechanisms of Folic Acid

While epidemiological data suggest a strong correlation between FA levels and the risk of NTDs, much of the scientific nature of this relationship remains unknown. The intracellular pathways of FA have been determined; however, the mechanisms leading to decreased risk for NTDs have not. Based on the current understanding of both FA and neural tube formation, different hypotheses are being studied in an effort to find the underlying mechanism.

FA functions intracellularly as a methylating agent. It provides the initial steps to several processes suspected to aid in the closure of the neural tube. Upon first entering the body, FA goes through a series of reactions to reach its activated form of 5-methyltetrahydrofolate (MTHF). This process synthesizes purines and thymidylate, both of which are critical for the processes of DNA replication and transcription (Beaudin *et al.*, 2007; Ross, 2010). After this progression, MTHF then enters the remethylation cycle, where it is utilized as a co-substrate in the methylation of homocysteine (HCY) to methionine (Martínez de Villarreal *et al.*, 2001). Evidence for this reaction includes an inverse relationship of FA and HCY, where low levels of FA correlate with a buildup of HCY (Richter *et al.*, 2001). As HCY is toxic to the cell, it must be removed. In the absence of adequate FA, HCY enters the transulfuration pathway, which converts the molecule to cystathionine in an irreversible reaction. While this does effectively rid the cell of a toxic substance, it also removes a source of cellular methionine, which significantly limits the ability of the remethylation cycle to proceed to the next steps (Beaudin *et al.*, 2007). In instances of adequate FA, methionine is produced, and enters the remethylation cycle. In this cycle, methionine is converted to *S*-adenosylmethionine (SAM), which is then converted to *S*-adenosylhomocysteine (SAH) after SAM acts to methylate several key intracellular components, including DNA, RNA, lipids, proteins, histones, and neurotransmitters (Beaudin *et al.*, 2007; Björklund *et al.*, 2006). In the cell, SAH acts through negative feedback to inhibit the enzymes required for SAM generation.

In order to limit this inhibition SAH must be removed through its conversion to HCY. This remethylation cycle can be seen in Figure 2. While the ratio of SAM/SAH has been measured at 4.6-6.9 in normal adult rat liver cells, the ratio can increase to 42 in the cells of a rat embryo. This indicates a significant increase in the demand for SAM in the development of an embryo as compared to a fully developed cell (Björklund *et al.*, 2006). In an environment with adequate FA intake, the increase in SAM can result from both an increased conversion of HCY to methionine and a decrease in the negative feedback of SAH resulting from the decreasing levels of HCY. In cases of FA deficiency, however, one study on mice found the SAM/SAH ratio to be significantly reduced in embryos with low FA intake, when compared to an embryo at the same developmental stage with a standard diet (Burren *et al.*, 2008). This evidence suggests that low FA levels limit the ability to generate SAM, allowing for improper development of the embryo.

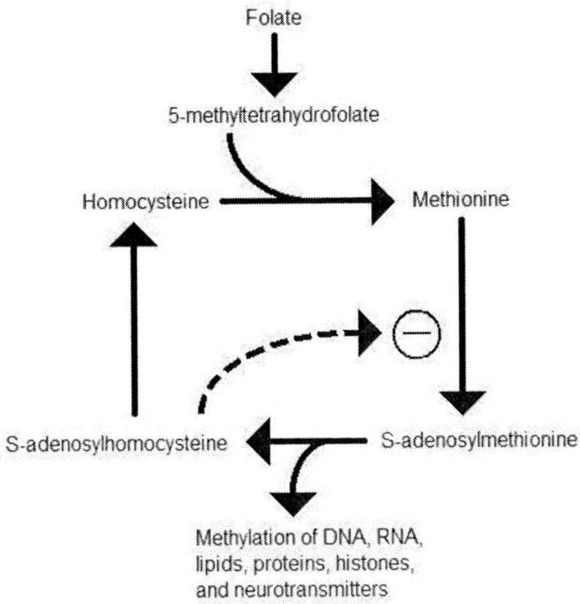

Figure 2. The intracellular remethylation cycle. FA is activated and acts as a co-substrate in the generation of methionine. Methionine is converted to SAM, the most important component of proper neural tube formation. Decreases in FA lead to a buildup of homocysteine and SAH, causing a decrease in the precursors to SAM and the activity of the enzymes that form SAM.

This chemical pathway and its relationship to the formation of NTDs have been confirmed through several studies. One such study on a Mexican population of women compared mothers with a NTD pregnancy and mothers with healthy offspring. Results determined that erythrocyte FA levels were less than 160 ng/ml in 75.6% of the NTD group as compared to 51.2% in the control group (Martínez de Villarreal *et al.*, 2001). A French study by Bunduki, *et al.*, corroborated these findings when the FA levels of fetal and maternal blood in cases of NTDs were compared to those with other birth defects. These results also revealed significantly decreased levels of both total FA, as well as methylated FA in the maternal red blood cells of the NTD experimental group. More importantly, they also displayed a reduced methylated FA to total FA ratio, indicating a problem in FA methylation (Bunduki *et al.*, 1995). All of these results can be seen in Table 2. Though differences in fetal levels were not significant, these tests were not conducted during the first trimester, likely missing the critical development of the neural tube. These findings provide evidence for two potential causes for the development of NTDs: a deficiency in FA and a decreased ability to methylate FA.

In order to more accurately understand this relationship, several additional studies have been conducted. One such study conducted by Lucock *et al.* in the United Kingdom compared non-pregnant women with a history of NTDs to a control group of non-pregnant women. Using blood samples, the levels of all FA intermediates of the methylation cycle were measured. As expected with a FA deficiency, this study found the experimental group to have significantly decreased levels of total erythrocyte FA. In addition to this, however, the NTD group also showed to have increases in serum HCY and the ratios of both HCY/tetrahydrofolate and HCY/vitamin B12. These numbers can be seen in Table 3. These results were indicative of a disturbance in the remethylation cycle. It was posited with these data that low FA levels may contribute to a problem involving vitamin B12, methionine synthase (MS), methylenetetrahydrofolate reductase (MTHFR), or a combination of these molecules, leading to an increased risk for an NTD (Lucock *et al.*, 1998). Given the importance of the remethylation cycle in the formation of SAM, it is suspected that the role of FA is to protect the developing embryo from problems arising from these three important cofactors.

Table 2. Significant results of study conducted by Bunduki *et al* measuring FA and methylated FA levels in maternal erythrocytes. These results exhibit decreased total levels and methylated levels in women with NTD pregnancies

	Experimental	Control	P-value
Total erythrocyte FA (ng/mL)	293.9	399.0	0.01
Methylated erythrocyte FA (ng/mL)	201.9	314.0	0.004
Methylated FA/Total FA	0.65	0.77	0.02

Table 3. Significant results of study conducted by Lucock *et al.* These results indicate a disturbance in the remethylation cycle due to low FA intake

	Experimental	Control	P-value
Total Erythroctye FA (ng/mL)	343	440	0.022
Serum HCY (µMol/L)	8.4	7.2	0.024
HCY/tetrahydrofolate	3.15	2.27	0.047
HCY/vitamin B12	0.023	0.017	0.016

One idea suggests that FA acts to counter the inhibitory role that nitric oxide (NO) has on MS. In rat studies, NO has been shown to induce NTDs through the process of MS inhibition. Thus, the methyl transfer from MTHF to HCY is inhibited. To further examine this principle Weil *et al.* conducted a study using chick embryos to investigate the effect of the addition of the NO donor *S*-nitroso-*N*-acetyl-penicillamine (SNAP) and FA on the incidence of NTDs. The results showed that of embryos between the eight and twelve somite stage placed in a high-SNAP environment, 70% had an open neural tube section, as opposed to only 24% of the untreated embryos. Groups treated either with only FA or with both SNAP and FA showed no statistical difference from the control group. To verify the activity of the NO in this experiment, hemoglobin was added to the SNAP group to quench the NO. This addition led to a significant reduction back to the baseline percentage of 22% open neural tube sections and thus provided some evidence for the role of NO in neural tube development. In order to determine its action on MS further tests were conducted. Using labeled methyl groups, MS activity was calculated between embryos with open and closed neural tubes. It was found that significantly higher levels of MS activity were present in the closed neural tube embryos, which consisted of the untreated and FA-treated groups. Upon further investigation of the open neural tube embryos, the addition of vitamin B12 was shown to significantly increase the activity of the MS (Weil *et al.*, 2004). The proposed mechanism behind this finding is that NO acts to sequester vitamin B12, a cofactor for MS. As FA intake increases, the effects of NO on B12 are decreased, thus returning activity to the MS enzyme.

Another area of study focused on a genetic component to the remethylation cycle. One critical enzyme in the process of activating MTHF for the generation of SAM is MTHFR. Within the gene coding for this enzyme, two polymorphisms have been shown to correlate with an increased risk of NTDs: *MTHFR* 677C to T and *MTHFR* 1298A to C (Richter *et al.*,

2001). A Martínez de Villarreal *et al.* study of Mexican women focused only on the *MTHFR* gene at nucleotide 677 and its relationship to NTD development. When comparing the genome of the NTD experimental and control groups, it was found that the experimental group's 39.5% frequency of the homozygous T/T gene was significantly greater than the control's frequency of 9.7%. Based on these results, a homozygous T/T mother had a relative risk of a NTD pregnancy of 6.1 as compared to the homozygous C/C and heterozygous genotypes (Martínez de Villarreal *et al.*, 2001). These findings strongly suggest the presence of a genetic predisposition to NTD development. As further research into this area of study, Richeter *et al.* conducted an experiment in Germany by examining both *MTHFR* polymorphisms and an insertion in the gene encoding cystathionine β-synthase (CBS), an enzyme that regulates HCY levels. The results of this study showed no significance for any of the three polymorphisms independently or for any relation to the *CBS* insertion. However there were significant results suggesting a relationship between the two *MTHFR* polymorphisms and neural tube defects. The frequency of being heterozygous at both nucleotides was found to be significantly greater in the experimental group (24.5%) as compared to the control group (16.3%). This was likely due to decreased MTHFR activity. Interestingly, of those who participated in the study there were no genotypes homozygous for both mutations, or homozygous for one mutation and also heterozygous for the other (Richter *et al.*, 2001). This suggests that these incidents of greater mutation would be insufficient to generate a viable embryo. Overall these findings indicate that the wild-type genes have a role in the closing of the neural tube, and that genetic abnormalities can lead to NTDs even in a state of adequate FA intake.

One study took this idea even further by suggesting that low FA intake was simply a risk factor for genetically predisposed individuals. Burren *et al.* based their study on the idea that although fortification efforts have shown the ability to reduce the incidence of NTDs, most affected pregnancies display maternal FA levels within the normal range. It was suggested that genetics do contribute to neural tube development within the FA methylation pathway. To test this, *splotch* ($Sp2^H$) mice carrying an intragenic deletion in the *Pax3* gene were fed a FA-deficient diet and compared to a standard diet control group. In these genetically predisposed mice, the NTD exencephaly occurred in 88% of the low-FA diet experimental group and only 61% of the standard diet control group. Likely related to this was the discovery that the FA-deficient embryos had 5.3 and 6.6 fewer somites during two different periods of development than that of the standard diet embryos. This evidence further strengthens the argument that while a genetic predisposition increases the risk for NTDs, an inadequate intake of FA can exacerbate the risk. Unfortunately, this study also demonstrated the absence of a significant difference in the methylation of cytosine, which had been a proposed mechanism for FA's role in neural tube development (Burren *et al.*, 2008). While relationships between FA and the remethylation cycle have been demonstrated, the mechanisms inducing NTDs still remain undefined. Differing hypotheses exist, but each focuses on the methylation of DNA, RNA, or proteins.

One possible hypothesis regarding FA's end role in neural tube development has been proposed by Björklund *et al.* and is based on the idea that the resulting increase in SAM causes an activation of the cytoskeleton required for neural cell differentiation. These increased levels are critical to the developing embryo because of the methylating actions of SAM on histidine and arginine. A recent study found that rat embryos grown in an environment of low methionine showed reductions of 56% and 42% in the methylated states of histidine and arginine, respectively. These two amino acids have been found to be highly conserved in the active sites of actin, myosin, α and β tubulin, and neurofilament L, each of which is methylated by SAM during neural tube closure. Assuming these pathways to be correct, a state of low FA and SAM would prevent the cytoskeletal elements of neural cells from localizing, thus limiting cell contraction and movement (Björklund *et al.*, 2006). This hypothesis suggests that adequate levels of FA would increase the amount of SAM available to the developing embryo. In turn, this would increase the ability of the neural tube to close and ultimately lower the risk of a NTD.

Another proposed hypothesis involves epigenetics. Beaudin *et al.* proposed that FA and the subsequent SAM are responsible for the gene silencing methylation reactions required for proper development. Adjacent cytosine and guanine nucleosides (CpG) can often be methylated within promoter regions to silence genes, which is believed to be critical for proper differentiation. One specific protein suspected to be silenced is in this process is histone deacetylase, which would ultimately increase the rates of replication and transcription in the developing embryo (Ross, 2010). As evidence for this proposal, embryos without the de novo methyltransferase enzymes required in this process have been shown to display NTDs. It is proposed that low levels of FA would also lead to this problem, by removing the source of the methyl group necessary for gene silencing. Overall, it is proposed that CpG-methylation alters the expression of up to 30% of the genome, which would be sufficient to effect the closure of the neural tube (Beaudin *et al.*, 2007).

Although neither the roles of cytoskeletal methylation nor gene silencing have been proven in neural tube development, they are one of many hypotheses based on the role of FA in the remethylation cycle. As our understanding of other factors – vitamin B12, the *MTHFR* gene, MS, and NO – evolves, the dietary levels of FA may need to be reviewed. As previously mentioned, excess FA is known to mask vitamin B12 deficiencies in some patients. In others, certain *MTHFR* alleles may increase the risk of NTDs above levels which can be reduced by FA. In order to ascertain the amount of FA that may be beneficial to reduce the risk of NTDs, it is necessary to continue researching the effects that FA has on all aspects of our physiological functions including diseased states.

Teratogenicity of Diabetes Mellitus Associated with Folic Acid Function

As one of the leading causes of death in the United States, diabetes mellitus and its complications must be taken into consideration when evaluating the risks of pregnancy. Offspring of women with pre-existing diabetes are at greater risk of a broad range of birth defects, of which NTDs and cardiovascular malformations are the most prevalent. The mechanisms by which those conditions occur are poorly understood, but studies have shown that FA supplementation can reduce the incidence of spina bifida and anencephaly (Williams *et al.*, 2002). Although proper blood glucose monitoring and insulin treatment have dramatically reduced the risk of birth defects in diabetic mothers, the incidence of NTDs is still two to six times that of non-diabetic mothers (Oyama *et al.*, 2008), indicating the need for better understanding of how diabetes affects the risk of NTDs in embryos.

Current research agrees that hyperglycemia acts as the primary teratogen in diabetic conditions. In 2001, Machado *et al.* studied the correlation between NTDs and alloxan (ALX)-induced diabetic hyperglycemia in heterozygous splotch (*Sp/+*) mice. Control mice did not receive ALX. Both treatment groups consisted of three genotypes with Sp received from either the mother or the father: +/+ x +/+, +/+ x *Sp/+*, and *Sp/+* x +/+. Embryos from ALX-treated mothers presented with decreased fetal weight and a marked increase in birth defects compared to controls. Incidents of exencephaly ranged from 14.6 ± 4.4% to 33.6% ± 6.2% across all three genotypes treated with ALX, yet it remained non-existent across all three genotypes in the controls. These results are depicted in Table 4. The presence of only one *Sp* gene more specifically correlated with increased incidence of exencephaly. Machado *et al.* demonstrated a strong correlation between hyperglycemia and a marked increase in malformations, especially in exencephaly and spina bifida. This paved the way for more in-depth study into how hyperglycemic conditions may induce malformations (Machado *et al.*, 2001).

Further exploring the connection between maternal diabetes and neural tube defects, Wentzel *et al.* determined that FA supplementation reduced the incidence of malformations while normalizing crown-to-rump length and somite count in rat embryos exposed to a diabetic or high-glucose environment. Embryos were exposed to either an *in vivo* diabetic environment in mothers with streptozotocin (STZ)-induced diabetes or an *in vitro* hyperglycemic environment (30 mM glucose). Compared to control mothers' embryos, exposure to a diabetic environment increased the incidence of NTDs in embryos from 4% to 71% *in vivo* and 0% to 88% *in vitro*. Subsequently injecting diabetic mothers with FA (15 mg/kg by daily subcutaneous injection beginning gestational day (GD) 0) lowered the incidence of *in vivo* NTDs to 3%, while administration of 1 mM and 2 mM of FA reduced the *in vitro* rate of NTDs to 29% and 5%, respectively, as shown in Table 5. Thus supplementation with FA reduced the incidence of NTDs caused by the diabetic/hyperglycemic environments (Wentzel *et al.*, 2005).

Wentzel *et al.* continued their research to show reduced mRNA expression for the FA transporter (folate-binding proteins, *Folbp*) in embryos exposed to the diabetic/hyperglycemic environments. Results showed a reduced FA concentration in the embryos on GD10. Knocking out either variant of *Folbp* (*Folbp-1* or *Folbp-2*) increased the incidence of NTDs. However, the lack of *Folbp-1* appeared to directly induce NTDs while null *Folbp-2* seemed to convey lesser FA transport inhibition by synergistically enhancing other teratogens' effects (Wentzel *et al.*, 2005). They postulated that diminished *Folbp*-mediated uptake of FA in the embryos would create a "state of functional FA deficiency" that could potentially be corrected by copious supplementation with exogenous FA (Wentzel *et al.*, 2005). Correlation between *Folbp* and embryonic FA concentration suggested a molecular mechanism by which diabetic hyperglycemia can mediate functional FA deficiency.

Table 4. Significant results of a study conducted by Machado *et al.* ALX treatment resulted in exencephaly in embryos across all three genotypes, compared to no incidence in same-genotype controls. The presence of a Sp gene, received from either the mother or the father, appeared to increase the incidence of exencephaly

	% of Exencephaly ± SEM	
	ALX (n)	Control (n)
+/+ x +/+	14.6 ± 5.0* (74)	0 (88)
+/+ x *Sp*/+	20.0 ± 4.4* (172)	0 (72)
Sp/+ x +/+	33.6 ± 6.2* (74)	0 (124)

* P≤0.05 compared with same-genotype controls

Table 5. Significant results of a study conducted by Wentzel *et al.* Folic acid supplementation reduced the incidence of open neural tube defects in rat embryos of mothers with STZ-induced diabetes *in vivo* and *in vitro*

		% of Open Neural Tubes in G11 Embryos (n)			
		No FA	FA (15	FA (1 mM)	FA (2 mM)
in vivo	N	4 (26)	0 (13)		
	STZ	71 (24)	3 (31)		
in vitro	N	0 (31)		N/A	0 (8)
	STZ	88 (34)		29 (14)	5 (21)

The beneficial effects of FA supplementation were corroborated by Oyama *et al.* in their study of the global effects of diabetes. External (most commonly exencephaly and spina bifida), cardiovascular, and skeletal malformations in addition to apoptosis of hindbrain cells were all elevated in embryos from mothers with STZ-induced diabetes as compared to controls. FA supplementation decreased the occurrence of all the above. The authors suggested that the observed increase in neuroepithelial apoptosis could contribute to aberrant neural tube closure and result in the NTDs. FA supplementation would help decrease the rate of apoptosis and thereby prevent the occurrence of NTDs (Oyama *et al.*, 2008). Further study by Gao and Gao demonstrated how the embryos of mice with STZ-induced diabetes showed decreased proliferation and increased apoptosis of neural progenitor cells that resulted in NTDs. The same effects were observed in embryos exposed *in vitro* to a hyperglycemic (30 mM glucose) environment (Gao and Gao, 2007). As previously described, a decreased ability of FA derivatives to participate in methylation reactions, DNA synthesis, and cell division can lead to the dysregulation of proper neural tube closure.

While FA deficiency often results from insufficient dietary intake by the mother, it can arise from an inability to transport FA across the placenta in less common instances. Since the fetus cannot synthesize its own FA it must rely on maternal intake and circulation. Transport of FA depends on placental FA receptors FRα and FRβ, reduced FA carrier 1 (RFC1), and proton-coupled FA transporter (PCFT). A study by Keating *et al.* examined how various pharmacological agents, recreational drugs, and pathological conditions interfered with normal FA uptake by the human syncytiotrophoblast. Human cytotrophoblasts (TB) were cultured and incubated with the various substances either acutely (26 minutes) or chronically (48 hours). TB cells are often used to model human placental transport and function, making them well suited for observing modulation of ^{3}H-FA uptake and cytotoxicity in this study. Neither acute nor chronic insulin exposure (50-5000 pM insulin acute, 50-500 pM chronic) affected ^{3}H-FA uptake or conferred any levels of cytotoxicity. Acute exposure to hyperglycemia (10-45 mM glucose) did not affect ^{3}H-FA uptake. However, chronic hyperglycemia (30 and 45 mM glucose) did inhibit ^{3}H-FA uptake by approximately 30%, dropping it to 70.9 ± 7.1% of control values. Furthermore, mRNA expression of FRα was reduced by 29% at hyperglycemic conditions (30 mM glucose). This suggested that chronic hyperglycemic conditions directly impact fetal ability to uptake FA at the cellular level (Keating *et al.*, 2009).

A diabetic or hyperglycemic environment can also lead to birth defects by promoting oxidative stress in both the mother and the fetus. FA can play a crucial role in attenuating, if not normalizing, the effects of oxidative stress. Wentzel and Eriksson investigated disturbances in the arachidonic cascade due to diabetic embryopathy, characterized by increased markers of oxidative stress *in vivo* and *in vitro*. Rat embryos from mothers with STZ-induced diabetes and those cultured in 30 mM glucose were analyzed to determine levels of isoprostanes, such as 8-epi-$PGF_{2\alpha}$, and prostaglandin E_2 (PGE_2). Isoprostanes and aberrant metabolism of PGE_2 both indicate peroxidation of arachidonic acid by nonenzymatic, free radical-catalyzed reactions, *i.e.*, lipid peroxidation. Controls for this study were embryos taken from nondiabetic mothers and those cultured in 10 mM glucose; all embryos were assessed approximately between GD10 and GD11. More malformations, especially NTDs, and decreased crown-to-rump length as well as somite number were found in embryos from diabetic environments compared to controls. Increased isoprostane concentration and decreased PGE_2 concentration compared to controls confirmed the increased level of oxidative stress in embryos from a diabetic milieu. Administration of dietary vitamin E *in vivo* and FA *in vitro* ameliorated all of the above parameters, suggesting that antioxidants (including FA) play an important role in normal embryonic development. Wentzel and Eriksson posit that a diabetic/hyperglycemic environment induces the overproduction of free radical oxygen species. This excess of free radicals leads to increased production of isoprostanes from arachidonic acid and decreased PGE_2 production, the latter of which requires arachidonic acid as a substrate. Excess free radicals and related species can impose oxidative stress to genetic material, resulting in increased teratogenicity and carcinogenicity. Here, antioxidants such as vitamin E and FA would act to quench the excess free radicals (Wentzel and Eriksson, 2005).

Gäreskog, Wentzel, and Eriksson further teased out the molecular effects of FA and vitamin E on apoptosis proteins in rat embryos *in vivo*. The group had noted that the intrinsic apoptosis pathway seemed to dominate the apoptotic mechanisms in diabetes-induced malformations and sought to evaluate its involvement through Western Blot analyses of two proteins, the antiapoptotic B-cell lymphoma 2 protein (Bcl-2) and the proapoptotic Bcl-2-associated x protein (Bax). Nuclear factor-κ B (NF-κB), a transcription factor capable of promoting the production of several antioxidative and antiapoptic proteins, was also measured by electromobility shift assays. Three treatment groups existed in addition to untreated normal and STZ-induced diabetic pregnant rats: (1) daily subcutaneous injections of 15 mg/kg FA dissolved in redistilled water beginning on GD0, (2) 5% dietary vitamin E supplementation, and (3) combination therapy of both supplements. In line with previous studies, increased frequency of malformations and decreased crown-to-rump length as well as somite numbers were found in embryos of diabetic mothers compared to controls. Decreased Bcl-2 and increased Bax protein levels were found in diabetic embryos, indicating a shift toward proapoptotic activity. FA and vitamin E treatment, both individually and together, led to some improvements in protein levels, but did not yield a consistent pattern of improvement across GD10 and GD11. No detectable levels of NF-κB activation was found in either diabetic or control embryos on GD10, but decreased activation of NF-κB in diabetic embryos was detected on GD 11, suggesting decreased antioxidative and antiapoptotic activity. FA supplementation and combined treatment both increased NF-κB in diabetic embryos. These findings support earlier claims that administration of antioxidant compounds can attenuate the negative effects of a hyperglycemic environment, particularly the rate of malformation and decreased NF-κB activation. The data further suggest that the dosage of each antioxidant, rather than their additive or synergistic effects, is crucial to optimizing protective effects, evidenced by their effects on Bcl-2 and Bax protein levels. Gareskog *et al.* concluded that both antioxidants acted on the same teratological processes to attenuate oxidative damage, which can lead to birth defects such as NTDs (Gäreskog *et al.*, 2006).

Zabihi *et al.* further examined the molecular and cellular effects of FA supplementation on oxidative stress, apoptosis, and vascular morphology. Analysis of protein levels and distributions in embryos from pregnant rats with STZ-induced diabetes showed increased levels of CuZn-superoxide dismutase (CuZnSOD) and an increased Bax/Bcl-2 ratio in the yolk sacs of diabetic embryos, indicating oxidative stress and increased apoptotic activity, respectively. Both imbalances were corrected with 15 mg/kg of FA supplementation via daily subcutaneous injection beginning from GD0. In addition, VEGF-A protein levels were decreased in diabetic embryos. Blood vessels of diabetic embryos in comparison with control embryos were fewer and smaller, and poorly organized. FA supplementation normalized both vascular conditions (Zabihi *et al.*, 2007).

Finally, Zúñiga-González *et al.* evaluated the effect of FA supplemention on the level of oxidative stress in STZ-diabetic rats and their embryos, using micronucleated species as markers of damage. Weekly blood samples from diabetic pregnant rat mothers and controls were tested for micronucleated polychromatic erythrocytes (MNPCEs) while their newborn pups were tested for micronucleated erythrocytes (MNEs) as well as MNCPEs. Diabetic mothers and their pups exhibited elevated levels of MNPCEs and MNEs in comparison with controls, but did not experience a significant decrease in levels with 0.7 mg/kg of daily FA supplementation via oral gavage. A parallel study with buccal mucosa samples from adult human subjects demonstrated increased levels of micronucleated cells (MNCs) in diabetic individuals that were significantly lowered after a 30-day regimen of 5 mg of FA per day ($P < 0.001$). Based on the results of the human study, the investigators surmised that the rats did not respond to FA treatment due either to the brevity or the insufficient dosage of the treatment schedule. Although the subjects of the human study were not pregnant, the results do indicate a significant role for FA in protecting against oxidative damage as measured by MNC levels (Zúñiga-González *et al.*, 2007).

These four studies suggest that FA plays an important role in keeping oxidative damage in check. Diabetes mellitus can overwhelm the system with excess free radical production and exacerbate any FA deficiency. This cascade can ultimately lead to oxidative damage and aberrant apoptosis as posited by Oyama *et al.* and Gao and Gao.

Recent research has elucidated many mechanisms by which diabetes mellitus may increase the risk of NTDs, drawing correlations between hyperglycemia, functional FA deficiency, oxidative stress, and cellular dysregulation of neural tube closure. However, the studies have indicated that the precise mechanisms are complex and interconnected, as summarized in Figure 3, warranting deeper investigation.

A report published in October 2010 by the Centers for Disease Control and Prevention, Division of Diabetes Translation, projected that the prevalence of diabetes mellitus in the US adult population would reach 25-28% by 2050. If the recent surge in incidences of diabetes continues coupled with low mortality, this statistic could climb to 33% (Boyle *et al.*, 2010). Bombard *et al.* also found that low-income and obese mothers were more likely to have three or more chronic diseases and/or related risk factors. Although the prevalence of pre-existing diabetes was low (<3%), low-income women still had almost twice the prevalence as higher-income women, putting them at greater risk for complications in pregnancy (Bombard, *et al.*, 2010). Even more worrisome, a 2007 study by Case *et al.* conducted in Texas found that diabetic women were less likely to know of the beneficial and protective effects of FA, while obese women were less likely to supplement with FA (Case *et al.*, 2007).

Diabetes mellitus is and will continue to be a major concern across all medical and health disciplines, calling for better understanding and control. Careful blood glucose monitoring, insulin treatment, adequate nutrition, and the use of multivitamins (including 400 μg/day of FA) (Center for Disease Control and Prevention) prior to conception will help reduce the risk of NTDs in pregnant women with pre-existing diabetes (Correa *et al.*, 2003). Yet there are physicians prescribing significantly higher doses of FA to try to offset the increased risk of congenital malformations. Capel and Corcoy question the safety and efficacy of such measures, noting that high levels of FA can aggravate vitamin B12 deficiency and promote neoplasia. In addition to molecular and cellular research, future studies must also investigate the dosage of FA that minimizes congenital malformations as well as toxicity for diabetic women (Capel and Corcoy, 2007). Despite the demonstrated effectiveness of FA supplementation when used in conjunction with insulin therapies, its interactions with other drugs may have risks for adverse effects.

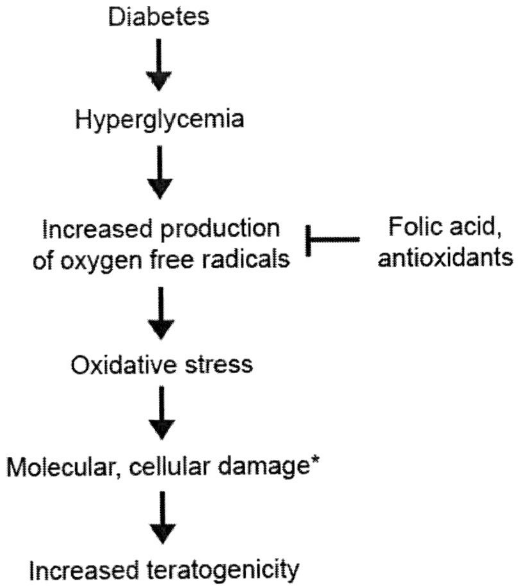

* Damage can include increased DNA breakage, micronuclei, lipid peroxidation, and altered levels of apoptotic proteins.

Figure 3. Possible mechanism of hyperglycemia-induced teratogenicity. Increased production of free radicals leads to a state of oxidative stress and damage that is manifested through many markers. Accumulated damage can lead to aberrant apoptosis, which is thought to be a major mechanism behind NTDs. Folic acid and other antioxidants help keep the production of free radicals in check, halting the progression of oxidative damage.

Folic Acid Supplementation in Pregnant Women with Epilepsy

While FA supplementation during pregnancy has been shown to provide substantial benefits in the general population, it presents complications for the care of pregnancy in women with epilepsy (WWE). Good seizure control throughout pregnancy is crucial for the safety of both mother and fetus (Robinson and Cleary-Goldman, 2008; Ornoy, 2009), yet the interaction of antiepileptic drugs (AEDs) and FA poses risks whose mechanisms remain unclear. For instance, FA supplementation appears to be less effective against NTDs in some WWE being treated with AEDs (Craig *et al.*, 1999; Yerby,

2003; Candito *et al.*, 2006; Smith, 2009). Some studies have demonstrated only a weak relationship between supplemental FA and protection against NTDs in fetuses of WWE treated with AEDs, suggesting that AEDs must affect other factors besides serum FA levels to induce NTDs (Morrow *et al.*, 2008). There is even some speculation that FA may exacerbate the onset of seizures (Guidolin *et al.*, 1998; Reynolds, 2002), though there is sparse evidence to support this. On the other hand, other studies have shown significant decreases in AED-induced NTDs in mice with perinatal FA treatment (Padmanabhan and Shafiullah, 2003; Dawson *et al.*, 2005).

When administered *in utero*, almost every AED has been associated with an increased risk – 4-6% overall, or twice that of the general population – of a range of fetal abnormalities, with exposure to higher doses (*e.g.*, > 1000 mg/day of VPA) resulting in a greater risk of being affected (Ornoy, 2009). A number of these include intrauterine growth retardation, congenital malformations, and cognitive dysfunction. While most AEDs do not display a particular pattern of abnormalities, there is a strong correlation between the use of valproic acid (VPA) or carbamazepine (CBZ) and the occurrence of NTDs (Yerby, 2003).

While the exact mechanism by which AEDs induce NTDs is unknown, several hypotheses exist. For instance, VPA is suspected of causing problems with neural tube development by interfering with FA absorption (Hendel, 1984) and metabolism (Yerby, 2003), or disrupting the methylation cycle by interfering with the conversion of methionine to SAM (Úbeda *et al.*, 2002). CBZ and phenobarbitone, which induce the drug-metabolizing enzyme cytochrome P450, have been shown to reduce serum FA levels significantly more than non-enzyme-inducing AEDs (Kishi *et al.*, 1997).

However, the protective effect of FA against NTDs is challenging to research because it appears to be strain-dependent in the mouse model. For instance, folate levels did not significantly correlate with the susceptibility of Folbp2KO mice to VPA-induced NTDs (Spiegelstein *et al.*, 2003). In the TO strain of mice, however, continuous dosing of FA throughout organogenesis has been shown to render significant protection ($p < 0.05$) against VPA-induced NTDs (Padmanabhan and Shafiullah, 2003). In another strain, the CD-1 mice, continuous dosing of FA was also shown to be effective against VPA-induced NTDs (Figure 4), as well as against alterations in the embryonic levels of the proteins p53, NF-κB, Pim-1, c-Myb, and Bax/Bcl-2. These results suggest that elevated FA levels throughout organogenesis may counteract the changes in FA distribution caused by VPA, thereby allowing complete neural tube closure through proper DNA and protein methylation, DNA synthesis, and maintenance of DNA integrity (Dawson *et al.*, 2005).

Because good seizure control before and during pregnancy is crucial for the protection of both mother and fetus, it is not possible to withhold AEDs for the duration of pregnancy. The severity of a patient's seizure disorder must first be assessed, and the drug regimen simplified as much as possible to minimize risk of teratogenicity (Robinson and Cleary-Goldman, 2008). However, as every individual metabolizes and reacts to drugs differently, it is inappropriate to designate any one AED as the "best" AED for pregnancy (Yerby, 2003). In cases where known teratogens such as VPA or CBZ cannot be avoided, it is the responsibility of the physician to prescribe the minimal dose necessary to prevent seizures, and encourage antenatal screening for NTDs.

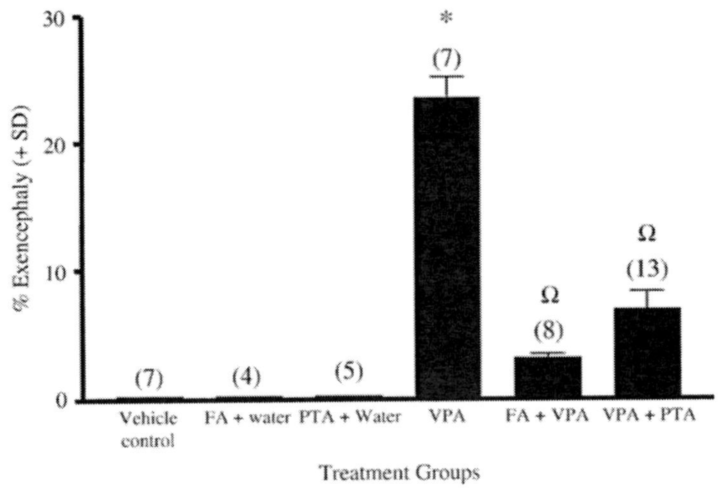

Figure 4. The effect of FA or pantothenic acid supplementation on VPA-induced NTDs in CD-1 mice. The protective effect of folic acid or pantothenic acid against VPA-induced exencephaly in CD-1 embryos was examined. In the FA studies, pregnant dams were treated with three doses of FA (4 mg/kg) per day on GDs 5-10 and VPA (0 or 400 mg/kg) on GD 9. For the pantothenic acid studies, pregnant dams were treated with three doses of pantothenic acid (3 x 200 mg/kg) and VPA (0 or 400 mg/kg) on GD 9. In both cases, animals were sacrifices on GD 19 and the fetuses were analyzed for exencephaly. Significant differences from the control group are indicated by * ($P<0.05$). Significant differences from the VPA alone treated groups are indicated by Ω ($P<0.05$). "*n*" values are indicated in parentheses on the appropriate bars, and represent the number of litters analyzed. Neural tube closure was measured as a rate (%) per treated litter. Figure used with permission from Dawson *et al.*, 2005.

Due to the early timing of organogenesis and neural tube closure, a WWE unaware of her pregnancy may miss the timing to adjust her AED regimen and FA intake in time to lower the risk of NTDs (Verrotti *et al.*, 2006; Ornoy, 2009). Thus it is imperative to educate WWE of the increased risks they carry and encourage better planning of their pregnancies. Though the evidence for FA supplementation against AED-induced NTDs is not yet definite, it is currently recommended that WWE planning a pregnancy adopt the higher periconceptual FA dosage of 4-5 mg/day. Given the interactions that AEDs can have on the effects of FA, it is critical to increase the intake beyond the normal recommendations for FA (Yerby, 2003; Verrotti *et al.*, 2006). Although this level of FA intake is significantly higher than that recommended during a healthy pregnancy, this represents just one of the many complications of pregnancy in a diseased state.

Conclusion

Although FA supplementation and fortification have dramatically reduced the rate of NTDs including spina bifida and anencephaly, NTD risk has not been fully eradicated. Current research suggests other factors exist in understanding and correcting FA deficiencies. The factors MTHFR, MS, NO, and vitamin B12 are all suspected to play a role in the development of the neural tube, given their contributions to the remethylation cycle. Defects in any of these factors have been shown to increase the risk for NTDs. FA supplementation has been critical in reducing the risks caused by these genetic predispositions and deficiencies.

In the condition of diabetes mellitus, these risks have been exacerbated, further necessitating the intake of FA. Hyperglycemic conditions have been shown to impair *Folbp*-mediated FA transport across the placenta as well as decrease proliferation and increase abnormal apoptosis of neural progenitor cells through oxidative damage to cells. FA supplementation is able to attenuate a significant portion of these risks, but NTD incidence for diabetic mothers is still two to six times that of non-diabetic mothers.

In women with epilepsy, patient education is crucial. This is due to the added risk of NTDs posed by the administration of AEDs, coupled with the timing of neural tube development early in gestation. WWE planning a pregnancy should be put on a higher periconceptual FA supplementation regimen of 4-5 mg/day, as well as the lowest possible dose of AEDs for preventing seizures.

While FA deficiency is certainly not the only risk factor for the development of NTDs, its ability to decrease risk further demonstrates the need to fortify foods with FA. Given this information it is critical for pregnant women to continue supplementation of FA, though additional research is certainly necessary to further develop understanding of these mechanisms. One such area of research to continue would be to pinpoint the end result of FA deficiency. Although cytoskeletal involvement has been hypothesized, it is clear that other mechanisms may be implicated. Determining these mechanisms may lead to the discovery of FA replacement therapies including treatments that coincide more appropriately with current diabetes mellitus and epilepsy therapies.

References

Amarin, ZO; Obeidat, AZ. Effect of folic acid fortification on the incidence of neural tube defects. *Paediatr. Perinat. Epidemiol.* 2010 Jul 1. 24(4):349-351.

Beaudin, AE; Stover, PJ. Folate-mediated one-carbon metabolism and neural tube defects: balancing genome synthesis and gene expression. *Birth Defects Res. C Embryo Today*. 2007. 81:183-203.

Björklund, NK; Gordon, R. A hypothesis linking low folate intake to neural tube defects due to failure of post-translation methylations of the cytoskeleton. *Int. J. Dev. Biol.* 2006. 50(2-3):135-141.

Bombard, JM; Dietz, PM; Galavotti, C; England, LJ; Tong, VT; Hayes, DK; Morrow, B. Chronic Diseases and Related Risk Factors among Low-Income Mothers. *Matern Child Health J.* 2010 Dec 14. [Epub ahead of print].

Boyle, JP; Thompson, TJ; Gregg, EW; Barker, LE; Williamson, DF. Projection of the year 2050 burden of diabetes in the US adult population: dynamic modeling of incidence, mortality, and prediabetes prevalence. *Popul Health Metr.* 2010 Oct 22. 8(1): 29.

Bunduki, V; Dommergues, M; Zittoun, J; Marquet, J; Muller, F; Dumez, Y. Maternal-fetal folate status and neural tube defects: A case control study. *Biol. Neonate.* 1995. 67(3):154-159.

Burren, KA; Savery, D; Massa, V; Kok, RM; Scott, JM; Blom, HJ; Copp, AJ; Greene, ND. Gene-environment interactions in the causation of neural tube defects: folate deficiency increases susceptibility conferred by loss of Pax3 function. *Hum. Mol. Genet.* 2008 Dec 1. 17(23):3675-3685.

Candito, M; Naimi, M; Boisson, C; Rudigoz, JC; Gaucherand, P; Guéant, JL; Luton, D; Van Obberghen, E. Plasma vitamin values and antiepileptic therapy: case reports of pregnancy outcomes affected by a neural tube defect. *Birth Defects Res. A Clin. Mol. Teratol.* 2007 Jan. 79(1):62-64.

Capel, I; Corcoy, R. What dose of folic acid should be used for pregnant diabetic women?. *Diabetes Care.* 2007 Jul. 30(7):e63.

Case, AP; Ramadhani, TA; Canfield, MA; Beverly, L; Wood, R. Folic acid supplementation among diabetic, overweight, or obese women of childbearing age. *JOGNN - Journal of Obstetric, Gynecologic, and Neonatal Nursing*. 2007 Jul-Aug. 36(4):335-341.

Center for Disease Control and Prevention http://www.cdc.gov/mmwr/ preview/mmwrhtml/mm5701a4.htm#fig Accessed 27 February 2011.

Chen, LT; Rivera, MA. The Costa Rican experience: reduction of neural tube defects following food fortification programs. *Nutr.Rev.* 2004 Jun. 62(6 Part 2):S40-3.

Correa, A; Botto, L; Liu, Y; Mulinare, J; Erickson, JD. Do multivitamin supplements attenuate the risk for diabetes-associated birth defects?. *Pediatrics.* 2003 May. 111(5 Part 2):1146-1151.

Craig, J; Morrison, P; Morrow, J; Patterson, V. Failure of periconceptual folic acid to prevent a neural tube defect in the offspring of a mother taking sodium valproate. *Seizure*. 1999 Jun. 8(4): 253-254.

Daly, S; Mills, JL; Molloy, AM; Conley, M; Lee, YJ; Kirke, PN; Weir, DG; Scott, JM. Minimum effective dose of folic acid for food fortification to prevent neural-tube defects. *Lancet.* 1997 Dec 7. 350(9092):1666-1669.

Dawson, JE; Raymond, AM; Winn, LM. Folic acid and pantothenic acid protection against valproic acid-induced neural tube defects in CD-1 mice. *Toxicol. Appl. Pharmacol.* 2006 Mar. 211(2):124-132.

De Steur, H., X. Gellynck, S. Storozhenko, G. Liqun, W. Lambert, D. Van Der Straeten, and J. Viaene. 2010. Health impact in China of folate-biofortified rice. *Nat.Biotechnol.* 28:554-556.

De Wals, P; Tairou, F; Van Allen, MI; Lowry, RB; Evans, JA; Van den Hof, MC; Crowley, M; Uh, SH; Zimmer, P; Sibbald, B; Fernandez, B; Lee, NS; Niyonsenga, T. Spina bifida before and after folic acid fortification in Canada. *Birth Defects Res. A Clin. Mol. Teratol.* 2008 Sep. 82(9):622-626.

Food Standards Agency http://www.eatwell.gov.uk/healthissues/factsbehindissues/folicacid/ Accessed 26 February 2011.

Gao, Q; Gao, YM. Hyperglycemic condition disturbs the proliferation and cell death of neural progenitors in mouse embryonic spinal cord. *Int. J. Dev. Neurosci.* 2007 Oct. 25(6):349-357.

Gäreskog, M; Eriksson, UJ; Wentzel, P. Combined supplementation of folic acid and vitamin E diminishes diabetes-induced embryotoxicity in rats. *Birth Defects Research.* 2006 Jun. 76(6):483-490.

Guidolin, L; Vignoli, A; Canger, R. Worsening in seizure frequency and severity in relation to folic acid administration. *Eur J Neurol.* 1998 May. 5(3):301-303.

Hendel, J; Dam, M; Gram, L; Winkel, P; Jørgensen, I. The effects of carbamazepine and valproate on folate metabolism in man. *Acta Neurol. Scand.* 1984 Apr. 69(4):226-231.

Hertrampf, E; Cortes, F. 2004. Folic acid fortification of wheat flour: Chile. *Nutr.Rev.* 62:S44-8.

Keating, E; Goncalves, P; Campos, I; Costa, F; Martel, F. Folic acid uptake by the human syncytiotrophoblast: interference by pharmacotherapy, drugs of abuse and pathological conditions. *Reprod. Toxicol.* 2009 Dec. 28(4):511-520.

Kishi, T; Fujita, N; Eguchi, T; Ueda, K. Mechanism for reduction of serum folate by antiepileptic drugs during prolonged therapy. *J. Neurol. Sci.* 1997 Jan. 145(1):109-112.

Lopez-Camelo, JS. Castilla EE. Orioli IM. INAGEMP (Instituto Nacional de Genetica Medica Populacional). ECLAMC (Estudio Colaborativo Latino Americano de Malformaciones Congenitas). 2010. Folic acid flour fortification: impact on the frequencies of 52 congenital anomaly types in three South American countries. *American Journal of Medical Genetics. Part A.* 152A:2444-2458.

Lucock, MD; Daskalakis, I; Lumb, CH; Schorah, CJ; Levene, MI. Impaired regeneration of monoglutamyl tetrahydrofolate leads to cellular folate depletion in mothers affected by a spina bifida pregnancy. *Mol. Genet. Metab.* 1998 Sep. 65(1):18-30.

Machado, AF; Zimmerman, EF; Hovland Jr, DN; Weiss, R; Collins, MD. Diabetic embryopathy in C57BL/6J mice. Altered fetal sex ratio and impact of the splotch allele. *Diabetes.* 2001 May. 50(5):1193-1199.

Martínez de Villarreal, LE; Delgado-Enciso, I; Valdez-Leal, R; Ortiz-Lopez, R; Rojas-Martinez, A; Limon-Benavides, C; Sanchez-Pena, MA; Ancer-Rodriguez, J; Barrera-Saldana, HA; Villarreal-Perez, JZ. Folate levels and

N(5),N(10)-methylenetetrahydrofolate reductase genotype (MTHFR) in mothers of offspring with neural tube defects: a case-control study. *Arch. Med. Res.* 2001 Jul-Aug. 32(4):277-282.

Morrow, JI; Hunt, SJ; Russell, AJ; Smithson, WH; Parsons, L; Robertson, I; Waddell, R; Irwin, B; Morrison, PJ; Craig, JJ. Folic acid use and major congenital malformations in offspring of women with epilepsy: a prospective study from the UK Epilepsy and Pregnancy Register. *J. Neurol. Neurosurg. Psychiatry.* 2009 May. 80(5):506-511.

Obican, SG; Finnell, RH; Mills, JL; Shaw, GM; Scialli, AR. 2010. Folic acid in early pregnancy: a public health success story. *FASEB Journal.* 24:4167-4174.

Oddy, WH; Miller, M; Payne, JM; Serna, P; Bower, CI. Awareness and consumption of folate-fortified foods by women of childbearing age in Western Australia. *Public Health Nutr.* 2007 Oct. 10(10):989-995.

Ornoy, A. Valproic acid in pregnancy: how much are we endangering the embryo and fetus?. *Reprod. Toxicol.* 2009 Jul. 28(1):1-10.

Oyama, K; Sugimura, Y; Murase, T; Uchida, A; Hayasaka, S; Oiso, Y; Murata, Y. Folic acid prevents congenital malformations in the offspring of diabetic mice. *Endocr. J.* 2009 Mar. 56(1):29-37.

Padmanabhan, R; Shafiullah, MM. Amelioration of sodium valproate-induced neural tube defects in mouse fetuses by maternal folic acid supplementation during gestation. *Congenit. Anom.* 2003 Mar. 43(1):29-40.

Reynolds, EH. Benefits and risks of folic acid to the nervous system. *J. Neurol. Neurosurg. Psychiatry.* 2002 May. 72(5):567-571.

Richter, B; Stegmann, K; Roper, B; Boddeker, I; Ngo, ET; Koch, MC. Interaction of folate and homocysteine pathway genotypes evaluated in susceptibility to neural tube defects (NTD) in a German population. *J. Hum. Genet.* 2001. 46(3):105-109.

Robinson, JN; Cleary-Goldman, J. Management of epilepsy and pregnancy: an obstetrical perspective. *Int. Rev. Neurobiol.* 2008. 83:273-282.

Ross, ME. Gene-environment interactions, folate metabolism and the embryonic nervous system. *Wiley Interdiscip. Rev. Syst. Biol. Med.* 2010. 2:471-480.

Sayed, AR; Bourne, D; Pattinson, R; Nixon, J; Henderson, B. 2008. Decline in the prevalence of neural tube defects following folic acid fortification and its cost-benefit in South Africa. *Birth Defects Research.* 82:211-216.

Smith, J; Whitehall, J. Sodium valproate and the fetus: a case study and review of the literature. *Neonatal Netw.* 2009 Nov-Dec. 28(6):363-367.

Spiegelstein, O; Merriweather, MY; Wicker, NJ; Finnell, RH. Valproate-induced neural tube defects in folate-binding protein-2 (Folbp2) knockout mice. *Birth Defects Res. Part A Clin. Mol. Teratol.* 2003 Dec. 67(12):974-975.

Úbeda, N; Alonso-Aperte, E; Varela-Moreiras, G. Acute valproate administration impairs methionine metabolism in rats. *J. Nutr.* 2002 Sep. 132(9):2737-2742.

Verrotti, A; Tana, M; Pelliccia, P; Chiarelli, F; Latini, G. Recent advances on neural tube defects with special reference to valproic acid. *Endocr. Metab. Immune Disord. Drug Targets.* 2006 Mar. 6(1):25-31.

Weil, M; Abeles, R; Nachmany, A; Gold, V; Michael, E. Folic acid rescues nitric oxide-induced neural tube closure defects. *Cell Death Differ.* 2004 Mar. 11(3):361-363.

Wentzel, P; Eriksson, UJ. A diabetes-like environment increases malformation rate and diminishes prostaglandin E(2) in rat embryos: reversal by administration of vitamin E and folic acid. *Birth Defects Research.* 2005 Jul. 73(7):506-511.

Wentzel, P; Gareskog, M; Eriksson, UJ. Folic acid supplementation diminishes diabetes- and glucose-induced dysmorphogenesis in rat embryos in vivo and in vitro. *Diabetes.* 2005 Feb. 54(2):546-553.

Williams, LJ; Mai, CT; Edmonds, LD; Shaw, GM; Kirby, RS; Hobbs, CA; Sever, LE; Miller, LA; Meaney, FJ; Levitt, M. Prevalence of spina bifida and anencephaly during the transition to mandatory folic acid fortification in the United States. *Teratology.* 2002 Jul. 66(1):33-39.

Yerby, MS. Clinical Care of Pregnant Women with Epilepsy: Neural Tube Defects and Folic Acid Supplementation. *Epilepsia.* 2003. 44(Suppl 3):33-40.

Zabihi, S; Eriksson, UJ; Wentzel, P. Folic acid supplementation affects ROS scavenging enzymes, enhances Vegf-A, and diminishes apoptotic state in yolk sacs of embryos of diabetic rats. *Reproductive Toxicology.* 2007 Jun. 23(4):486-498.

Zúñiga-González, GM; Batista-González, CM; Gómez-Meda, BC; Ramos-Ibarra, ML; Zamora-Perez, AL; Muñoz-Magallanes, T; Ramos-Valdés, C; Gallegos-Arreola, MP. Micronuclei in diabetes: folate supplementation diminishes micronuclei in diabetic patients but not in an animal model. *Mutation Research.* 2007 Dec 1. 634(1-2):126-134.

In: Folic Acid
Editors: Mária Szabó and Eve Varga
ISBN: 978-1-62100-867-5

Chapter V

Folic Acid Every Day: Educational Campaign Promoted Knowledge Gain and Behavior Change

Kimberly Beauchamp and Julie Garden-Robinson
North Dakota State University, Fargo, North Dakota, US

Abstract

In a concerted effort, a statewide coalition educated women of childbearing age about the relationship between folic acid consumption and the risk of neural tube birth defects (NTDs) among infants. Whether a pregnancy is planned or unplanned, research indicates that timely folic acid intake among women can reduce the risk of having an NTD-affected pregnancy. According to the Centers for Disease Control and Prevention (CDC), consumption of folic acid, a B vitamin, may reduce a woman's NTD-risk by up to 70% if the vitamin is taken 30 days prior to conception and every day throughout pregnancy. The United States Public Health Service (USPHS) recommends that women of childbearing age consume 400 micrograms of folic acid every day and notes that special situations may require higher intake levels.

A university extension service and a Folic Acid/Health Pregnancy Task Force formed a strategic statewide coalition to promote the "Folic Acid Every Day" message through media, classes, and health fairs using CDC- and locally-developed resources. The message was promoted by more than 131 coalition partners including: the National Folic Acid Council, a medical foundation, the state chapter of the March of Dimes, Extension agents, regional Women, Infants and Children (WIC) staff, Public Health staff, commodity groups, franchise restaurants, and pharmacies. Using feedback from task force members, a communication-based intervention campaign was developed and modeled after the CDC's *Ready or Not* campaign. Coalition members administered a baseline survey (n=422), conducted a folic-acid education intervention, and administered a second survey (n=349) following the intervention.

Thousands of people were reached with folic acid information through the use of mass media advertising including radio public service announcements, bathroom stall ads, a statewide radio program, and newspaper columns. The folic acid message was promoted through newspaper columns, e-mail blasts, press releases, and a Web site. Additionally, the coalition promoted and distributed the folic acid message on a variety of materials including recipe cards, educational DVDs, brochures, posters, congratulations cards provided with marriage licenses, oral contraceptive packet auxiliary labels, and restaurant and grocery store coupons.

Following the intervention, folic acid awareness, knowledge, and supplement intake behavior increased among women of childbearing age. About 76% of the survey participants were aware of folic acid (up 1% from Survey One; $p > .05$), 65% were able to identify folic acid as a B vitamin (up 12% from Survey One; $p < .05$), 79% recognized the association between folic acid and NTDs (up 10% from Survey One; $p < .05$), and 45% were aware of the daily folic acid intake recommendation of 400 mcg (up 18% from Survey One; $p < .05$). Approximately 46% of the participants were able to identify that women of childbearing age should take folic acid prior to and during pregnancy (up 14% from Survey One; $p < .05$), and 58% of the participants were taking folic acid every day (up 17% from Survey One; $p < .05$). The follow-up survey results indicated that task force members raised folic acid awareness and knowledge among women within 63% of the state's counties, including the most populous cities. In conclusion, an effective folic acid education campaign may serve to reduce the number of females at risk for having an NTD-affected pregnancy during childbearing age, and this project may serve as a model for other state coalitions.

Keywords: Folic acid, women, educational campaign, coalition.

Introduction

Structural defects of the spinal cord and brain occur in the developing fetus within the first month following conception (CDC, 1992, para. 7), often before a woman realizes she is pregnant and long before her first prenatal visit (CDC, 1992, para. 13; CDC, 2001, para. 1). According to the U.S. Preventive Services Task Force (2009), about one in every 1000 births in the U.S. each year is affected by a neural tube birth defect (NTD) such as anencephaly or spina bifida (para. 13). An estimated 50-75% of NTDs are preventable through adequate intakes of folic acid (pteroylmonoglutamic acid) before and during the first trimester of pregnancy (CDC, 1999a, para. 1). Based on a synthesis of information from several studies, including those which used multivitamins containing folic acid at a daily dose level greater than or equal to 400 micrograms (mcg), public health experts concluded that folic acid at levels of 400 mcg per day will reduce the risk of NTDs (CDC, 1992, para. 5).

According to the CDC (1999b), more than 75% of women are unaware that they need folic acid before and during the first weeks of pregnancy (para. 3). Because adequate folic acid levels are required during the first 28 to 30 days of gestation, prior to closure of the neural tube, it is often too late to begin vitamin supplementation once pregnancy is confirmed (Bentley, Ferrini, & Hill, 1999, p.264). Whether a pregnancy is planned or unplanned, research shows that timely folic acid intervention reduces the risk of having an NTD-affected pregnancy.

Folic Acid

Folic acid, a B vitamin, is a synthetic compound used in fortified food and dietary supplements (Committee on Genetics, 1999, p. 325). Folic acid has been added to foods such as enriched breads, pastas, rice, fortified cereals, and vitamin supplements. For more than 20 years, most multivitamin preparations in the United States have contained 400 mcg of folic acid per serving (Oakley, 2007, p. 368). Research findings indicate that most women of childbearing age do not consume the recommended amount of folic acid on a daily basis (Hammond, Squires, &Treiman, 2000, p. 1).

Because not all women receive adequate levels of folic acid from the food supply, increasing the use of vitamins containing folic acid remains a significant component of NTD prevention (CDC, 2004, para. 1). While most supplement pills contain 400 mcg per pill (Mason, 2009, p. 209), an estimated 35 percent of the U.S. adult population regularly consumes a multivitamin supplement containing folic acid (Radimer et al., 2004, p. 341). In 1992, in an attempt to reduce the frequency of NTDs and their associated economic burden, the U.S. Public Health Service began to urge women of childbearing age in the United States to meet the daily folic acid intake recommendation of 400 mcg.

National Efforts

The CDC determined that an educational campaign was needed to inform the public about the relationship between folic acid and neural tube birth defects. In 1998, the National Council on Folic Acid (NCFA) and the *Ready or Not* campaign were created in response to this need. Through the *Ready or Not* campaign, the NCFA coalition, comprised of national organizations, health professional associations, nonprofit organizations, community health coalitions, state folic acid councils, and government agencies, aimed to improve health through the promotion of folic acid consumption benefits (Hammond et al., 2000, p. 2). Launched in May 1999, the *Ready or Not* campaign utilized radio, television, print public service announcements (PSAs), news coverage, and a range of mass media and support materials disseminated by coalition partners to reach women of childbearing age (Hammond et al., 2000, p. 2). Campaign objectives were selected to target specific knowledge, attitude, and/or behavior relative to folic acid among women of childbearing age (Hammond et al., 2000, p. 4).

Statewide Efforts

The present study utilized collaborative efforts of a coalition task force to implement a public health campaign modeled after the CDC's *Ready or Not* campaign. The overall campaign objectives were to increase folic acid awareness, knowledge and intake behavior among women of childbearing age. In order to evaluate communication effectiveness, the campaign objectives were established as:

- Following the intervention, folic acid awareness among female participants will increase to at least 50%.

- Following the intervention, folic acid knowledge among female participants will increase to at least 50%.
- Following the intervention, self-reported folic acid intake through supplementation among female participants will be greater than 25%.
- Following the intervention and data analysis, educator feedback will help determine gaps in folic-acid related discussions between service providers and clients, and contribute to the development of best practices for folic-acid and NTD communication.

Through the efforts of the statewide task force, folic acid education materials (including CDC materials) were distributed to women of childbearing age, using mass media and interpersonal channels. Mass media channels play a crucial role in the diffusion of a public health campaign. The role of interpersonal channels is especially useful in persuading an individual to adopt a new idea (Rogers, 2003, p. 205).

Best Practices in Communication

Communication effectiveness is an essential element of public health education campaigns and can make or break the success of prevention efforts. *Effectiveness* is the degree to which an intervention program fulfills its objectives (Rogers, 2003, p. 367). Rofail et al. (2011) pointed out that many factors contributed to the success of folic acid public health campaigns, including the identification of target groups not currently reached by existing campaigns, and the need to adapt campaigns to reach those hard-to-reach groups.

Risk messages can be designed to warn individuals about the potentiality of an unwanted, but possible event. Public health campaigns often promote risk-centered messages that forewarn the public of negative consequences that are linked to unhealthy behavior. However, as Sellnow, Ulmer, Seeger, and Littlefield (2009) pointed out, exposure to information does not automatically translate into an individual's level of understanding (p. 9). To reduce risk, a level of understanding of the message and potential risk needs to be ascertained, and eventually acted upon.

Industry leaders identify processes, practices and systems among organizations as "best practices." According to Seeger (2006), best practices "usually take the form of a general set of standards, guidelines, norms, reference points or benchmarks that inform practice and are designed to improve performance" (p. 233). The best practices drawn from lessons learned provide models for similar organizations. These practices commonly serve as a guide for communicating risk to the public. A risk, according to Heath (2006), is an occurrence that can have positive or negative consequences of varying magnitudes, the occurrence of which and the effects of which can be variously predicted, controlled, and harmful or beneficial (p. 245).

Conceptual Framework

Diffusion of innovation is a conceptual framework that can be used to explore how publics understand and respond to the USPHS folic acid recommendation. Everett Rogers is credited with the development of the conceptual paradigm *Diffusion of Innovation* (Berger, 2005). Early application of the diffusion model to U.S. agriculture began in the 1950s and has since been generalized to multiple fields, including public health (Rogers, 2004, p. 13). Because diffusion is concerned with the dissemination of messages among publics, the diffusion framework is of great value to many disciplines, especially the field of public health where the priority is to promote and maintain the well-being of a community or population (Haider & Kreps, 2004, p. 6).

The main elements in the diffusion of new ideas are defined as: (1) an *innovation* (2) that is *communicated* (3) *over time* (4) among the members of a *social system* (Rogers, 2003, p. 36). Because innovations are a type of communication message with effects that are relatively easy to isolate, diffusion research offers a useful theoretical framework through which to ascertain an understanding of change (Rogers, 2003, p. 104). Diffusion researchers often use Rogers' (2003) general model to investigate the timing of decisions made by individuals or systems choosing to adopt or reject new ideas, products, or behaviors. "The significant role that the diffusion of innovation can perform in health promotion efforts cannot be underestimated, especially with the use of mass media channels of communication to influence health awareness, education, decisions, practices, and care" (Haider & Kreps, 2004, p.6).

Change Agents

Change agents are individuals who influence the direction of their client's willingness to adopt or reject an innovation (Rogers, 2003, p. 366). A change agent often utilizes face-to-face-exchange to communicate with clients. The agricultural extension service is reported to be one of the world's most successful change agencies (Rogers, 2003. p. 391). The agricultural extension model consists of three main components: a research subsystem, county extension agents, and state extension specialists. In the capacity of change agents, county extension agents work with individuals at the local level (Rogers, 2003, p. 165).

Change agents are able to shape the consequences of an innovation through client interaction. Usually, change agents typically do not concentrate their efforts on their most disadvantaged clients, and many change agents do not try to contact their needier, lower-status clients because they think that their lower-status clients will not respond to the innovation diffusion efforts (Rogers, 2003, p. 383). Rather, change agents prefer contact with better educated, higher status individuals in a system, which in turn tends to widen socioeconomic gaps through the innovation diffusion process while decreasing the degree of equality in a social system (Rogers, 2003, p. 456). Socioeconomic elites are considered more responsive to suggested health behavior changes because they are said to have greater health knowledge to build on, and care more about themselves than individuals of lower socioeconomic status (Freimuth, 1995). This type of client stereotyping discourages contact initiation from change agents to the less disadvantaged clients (Rogers, 2003, p. 383). The present study utilized agencies and programs to specifically reach out to low-income audiences at risk for having an NTD-affected pregnancy, by targeting individuals who utilize public services such as food and nutrition programs, public health clinics, and the Women Infant and Children (WIC) programs. Clients enrolled in these programs must first meet low-income eligibility requirements.

Vulnerability

Low-income audiences are frequently at high risk for many health problems, and often are considered difficult to reach during campaign implementation (Freimuth, 1995). For example, low-income females of childbearing age who have not adopted the recommendation to consume 400 mcg of folic acid every day may be considered hard-to-reach. Lower educated and lower status individuals often are labeled "hard-to-reach" because they have not adopted behavior change strategies at the rate of their "counterpart elites" (Freimuth, 1995). For example, a service provider could consider female clients who never graduated from high school and who do not consume

400 mcg of folic acid every day as "hard to reach" and at risk for having an NTD-affected pregnancy. In comparison, a service provider may not label female clients who have graduated from high school and who do take a daily supplement containing folic acid as "hard-to-reach" because they are meeting the USPHS recommendation.

"Low income individuals often are depicted as both financially and psychologically impoverished, focused on short-term rewards, and therefore uninterested in pursuing preventative health benefits" (Freimuth, 1995). Due to lack of funds and inadequate nutrition, the health status of low income individuals, including women of childbearing age, may be compromised. When campaigns are evaluated for effectiveness, these groups of individuals typically emerge as less exposed, less knowledgeable, and less likely to change their behaviors (Freimuth, 1995).

Extension Family and Nutrition Program

The Family Nutrition Program (FNP) is a federally funded program that seeks to help families with limited incomes use available resources to improve food and nutrition practices in order to prevent nutrition-related health problems (Hoover, Martin, & Litchfield, 2009, p. 1). "The FNP is a free and voluntary educational program that teaches basic nutrition, food safety, preparation, food resource management, and food purchasing to individuals who are receive and who are eligible to receive food stamps" (Steinhaus, Brunt, Pankow, Garden-Robinson, & Terbizan, 2009, p. 2). For example, FNP service providers could teach clients the relationship between folate-rich foods and NTD-prevention.

Women Infants Children Program

The WIC program is a nutrition program administered at the federal level by the USDA's Food and Nutrition Service (FNS). In order to qualify for the WIC program, applicants must be considered at nutritional risk and they must meet income guidelines. Applicants are asked to fill out a diet and medical history and provide documentation that their family income does not exceed 185% of the federal poverty guidelines (WIC, 2009).

The mission of WIC is to safeguard the health of low-income families, including pregnant and breastfeeding women, infants and young children who are at nutritional risk. The program provides foods, nutrition information, health screenings, counseling and support to eligible clients (WIC, 2009). For example, the WIC service providers could screen clients for habits of daily folic acid consumption and provide information to those who are unaware of the relationship between folic acid intake and NTD-risk.

Public Health

Public Health offers family planning services to low-income clients, among its many roles. Public health clients often are enrolled in Medicaid and Medicare plans. Public health clinicians often provide education about reproduction to clients, including women of childbearing age who are trying to prevent pregnancy or seek a pregnancy (North Dakota Public Health [NDPH], 2009). For example, during physical exams, public health service providers could educate their clients about the USPHS recommendation to prevent NTDs and encourage clients to consume a folic acid-containing supplement every day.

Methods

A coalition-driven campaign was carried out through four phases: (1) task force member recruitment, (2) baseline survey administration, (3) education intervention, and (4) post-test survey administration. The goal of Phase One was to develop strategic partnerships to guide campaign development. Phase Two aimed to assess baseline folic acid awareness, knowledge, and behavior among women of childbearing age. During Phase Three, campaign efforts focused on the dissemination of folic acid education materials. Following the education intervention, Phase Four focused on measuring changes in folic acid awareness, knowledge, and behavior among women of childbearing age and soliciting feedback from the coalition partners.

Project Collaborators

In 2008, the university extension service and a statewide Folic Acid/Health Pregnancy Task Force formed a coalition to educate women of childbearing age about reducing the risk of NTDs through daily folic acid intake. This strategic coalition of partners and/or sponsors included: (1) 36 extension agents, (2) nine multicounty women, infants and children (WIC) program staff, (3) eight public health staff, (4) six grocery stores, (5) 23 restaurants, (6) 55 pharmacies, (7) two commodity groups, (8) the March of Dimes (MOD), (9) the NCFA (Spina Bifida Association), and (10) a medical foundation. A university extension food and nutrition specialist provided the leadership for the study, and a graduate student served as the project coordinator. Project collaborators were initially recruited through email Listserv provided by the university extension food and nutrition specialist. Additional collaborators were recruited through personal contacts and referrals from task force members.

Education Intervention

Conference calls and e-mails were used to inform task force members before and during the campaign. In a concerted effort, the task force coalition conducted a communication-based intervention campaign to educate North Dakotans about the relationship between folic acid intake and neural tube birth defects. Internet, telephone, radio, newspapers, and face-to-face communication methods were used to disseminate the USPHS message among women of childbearing age. A Web site served as a folic acid education resource for task force members and women of childbearing age. The educational intervention, using CDC and locally developed materials, took place between December 1, 2008 and February 15, 2009.

Grant funding and in-kind sponsorships were obtained for the purpose of paying the costs associated with mass media advertising, acquisition of promotional materials such as posters, emery boards and marriage certificate cards for community dissemination, auxiliary labels for pharmacy dissemination, and incentive materials for survey participants. Service providers from WIC and public health were asked to order and acquire the available *Ready or Not* education intervention materials directly from the CDC. The CDC materials for statewide extension agents were obtained and disseminated by the university extension specialist.

A Web site (www.ndsu.edu/health) was updated to market the campaign message and included links to folic acid-related information. Mass media distribution in four major cities across the state included radio PSAs and bathroom poster ads placed in retail establishments. Face-to-face methods of contact were utilized for community distribution of educational materials and surveys. University student interns placed brochures and posters throughout dining centers, and conducted health fairs to promote the USPHS recommendation to students and the general public. Thus, the coalition utilized Internet, telephone, community distribution, radio, newspapers, and face-to-face methods to market the folic acid awareness program.

Folic Acid Education Materials

A folic acid message was promoted through a variety of means to educate women of childbearing age on the USPHS daily recommendation. Thirty-four paid bathroom stall ads promoting the folic acid message were placed in movie theatres, coffee shops, restaurants, spas, bowling alleys, health clubs, and college hot spots. Using *Ready or Not* PSAs from the CDC, 154 radio spots were placed on nine popular statewide radio stations. The university extension specialist appeared as a guest on a statewide radio program, talking about folic acid benefits, and statewide extension agents used coalition materials in their media work, including newspaper columns and radio interviews. Throughout the state, coalition members distributed print materials listing folic acid messages. Print materials included recipe cards (14,000), educational DVDs (150), "Marriage Congratulation" cards (5,000), brochures (6,500), posters (900), information sheets (2,400), handouts (6,000), bookmarks (9,000), salon emery board/nail files (12,000), labels on oral contraceptive packets (55,000), table tents (55), grocery store bread coupons (2,000), restaurant orange juice coupons (2,000), pharmacy coupons for vitamins containing folic acid (2,000), and two folic acid-related news columns that ran in 40 state and regional newspapers and on Web sites.

Online distribution of the folic acid messages was used with the potential to reach thousands more women of childbearing age, and included: columns in online newspapers, e-mail blasts, and press releases to news outlets. Additionally, folic acid lesson plans and PowerPoint modules were publicly available for use by educators at the Web site www.ndsu.edu/health.

Measures

For Surveys One and Two, *awareness* was measured by an individual's response of having heard, read or seen anything about folic acid. Questions pertaining to folic acid awareness varied slightly between the two surveys. To evaluate an individual's level of folic acid awareness, Survey One participants were asked to respond to the following question: "Have you ever heard, read or seen anything about folic acid or folate?" To evaluate an individual's level of folic acid awareness, Survey Two participants were asked to respond to the following question: "In the past two months, where have you seen or heard information about folic acid or folate?"

Questions on Surveys One and Two were designed to measure an individual's knowledge of the USPHS folic acid recommendation. All survey participants were asked to respond to the following five questions:

1. What is folic acid or folate?
2. What are some sources of folic acid or folate?
3. Some health experts recommend that women get the recommended amount of folic acid/folate to ____________.
4. How much folic acid/folate is recommended daily for women during childbearing age?
5. During childbearing age, when should women take folic acid?

Survey questions that measured folic acid supplementation behavior varied slightly between Surveys One and Two. Survey One participants were asked to respond to the following question: "Do you take a pill containing folic acid on a "daily basis?" Survey Two respondents were asked to report how long they have been taking a daily vitamin or supplement containing folic acid, and selected from answer options of "I do not take one," "less than a month," or "more than a month."

Survey questions on Survey Three were designed to measure perceived folic acid and NTD communication between service providers and clients. As a measure of communication interaction, service providers were asked to respond questions such as, "Does your agency provide a script and/or checklist for you to follow, during a routine client visit that includes the mention of folic acid?"

Service providers were also asked whether or not they initiated discussions with clients about timely and adequate folic acid intake and neural tube birth defects. Perceived frequencies of folic acid discussions were also measured by asking participants to respond to questions such as, "How often do you typically bring up in discussion, the topic of folic acid and neural tube birth defects?" One question was designed to assess service providers' awareness of NTD-affected pregnancies among their clients.

Survey Instruments

Three survey instruments were developed for this project. Surveys One and Two were administered to the general population and clients of service providers. Survey Three was administered to service providers. Prior to data collection, the survey instrument protocols were submitted to the university's Institutional Review Board (IRB), and permission to conduct research with human subjects was granted.

Instrument Development

Surveys One and Two. Questions on Surveys One and Two were designed to gather demographic data of participants, and to provide an assessment of folic acid awareness, knowledge, and supplement intake behavior prior to and following the campaign. Additionally, the service provider of each participant was tracked. The USPHS folic acid recommendation was used to frame the survey questions, and questions were modeled after previously used MOD survey instruments. The questions in the present study were comparable to questions noted in previous MOD's publications for the CDC.

Survey Three. Questions on Survey Three were designed to: (1) gather demographic data of service providers, (2) provide an assessment of folic acid and NTD communication between service providers and clients, and (3) assess the service providers' awareness of clients who have had NTD-affected pregnancies.

Two faculty members who specialize in survey development, along with the statewide survey team, reviewed the survey questions for all three surveys. The survey instruments were revised based on their feedback. Survey materials were photocopied and provided in packets to coalition members to facilitate their data collection, and data were entered and analyzed at one central location.

Surveys

Surveys One and Two. Identical (or similarly worded) questions were included on Surveys One and Two so that comparative assessments could be drawn from participant responses. Although identifying information was not collected from participants, the IRB protocol allowed for the collection of general demographic data (e.g. age, gender, race, ethnicity, and proximity).

Data from Survey One were compared with data from Survey Two in order to determine changes in folic acid awareness, knowledge, and supplement behavior among female clients of service providers, following an educational intervention.

Survey One included 16 multiple-choice and fill-in-the-blank questions. Overall, survey questions were designed to gather general demographic data and provide insight into a baseline assessment of folic acid awareness, understanding, behavior, and associated risks among the target group prior to an educational intervention. The survey included five questions pertaining to demographic data including age, gender, ethnicity, race and county of residence. Respondents answered eight questions related to folic acid awareness and knowledge and three questions related to supplement intake behavior.

Survey Two included sixteen multiple choice and fill-in-the-blank questions. Overall, the questions were designed to gather general demographic data and provide insight into the changes in awareness, understanding, behavior, and associated risks among women of childbearing age, following the educational intervention. Respondents answered five questions pertaining to demographic data, including age, gender, ethnicity, race and county of residence, and six questions related to knowledge and awareness. Additionally, the survey included four questions related to folic acid knowledge and supplement behavior.

Survey Three was administered to service providers through Survey Monkey (an online survey tool). Overall, the questions were designed to gather general demographic data and provide insight into folic acid and NTD-discussions between service providers and clients. Respondents answered one question pertaining to service affiliation and five multiple-choice questions pertaining to communication tendencies.

Procedures

Survey One and Two participants were recruited by survey coordinators positioned at statewide service provider locations. The surveys were not necessarily administered to the same participants, so differences in folic acid awareness, knowledge, and behavior are not compared for changes at the individual level for Surveys One and Two. The university IRB did not allow for the collection of identifiable data. The convenience samples of survey respondents included low-income clients from extension FNP, WIC, and public health programs. Additional participants were drawn from statewide universities and community colleges. Surveys also were administered to the general public at health fairs, and wellness centers. Project collaborators were invited through a Listserv email invitation to respond to Survey Three.

Survey Administration

Survey packets for Surveys One and Two were distributed to 39 trained survey administrators positioned around the state. Each packet included instructions, an IRB-approved recruitment script and information sheet, survey questionnaires, and incentive "goodie" bags for each participant. Before each survey could be administered, voluntary participant consent was needed. Upon receiving verbal consent from participants, task force members administered the statewide surveys to participants and distributed goodie bags upon questionnaire completion. Each goodie bag contained promotional materials with a folic acid message, including recipe cards, coupons, bookmarks, key chains, and pencils. Each respondent spent approximately 10 minutes completing the survey. An online link to Survey Three was distributed via electronic mail to service providers positioned around the state, and the online survey took approximately 10 minutes to complete.

Data Collection

The data collection process for Surveys One and Two began in October 2008 and was completed in April 2009. Survey administration took place over two distinct periods. Survey Period One covered the time frame October 1, 2008 through December 31, 2008. Survey Period Two covered the time frame January 16, 2009 through April 1, 2009. The data collection process for Survey Three began on October 27, 2009 and was completed by November 23, 2009.

Data Analysis

Statistical analyses of all three surveys were conducted using SPSS statistical software (Statistical Package for the Social Sciences 17 for

Windows, Rel. 17.0.0, 2008; SPSS Inc. Chicago, IL, USA). Descriptive statistics were used to describe the demographic characteristics of the study participants and survey item responses. Cross-tabulations were used to examine the relationships and percentages of responses within groupings. Using a 95% confidence interval, unpaired data from Surveys One and Two were analyzed using the Z-approximation test for equality of two independent proportions.

Results

Descriptive Statistics

Of the Survey One participants, 83.3% were white, 13% were American Indian or Alaska Native, 2.1% were Asian, 0.9% were black, and 0.7% were Native Hawaiian or Other Pacific Islander. Of the Survey Two participants, 86.4% were white, 10.9% were American Indian or Alaska Native, 1.2% were Native Hawaiian or Other Pacific Islander, 0.9% were black, and 0.6% were Asian. The samples are representative of the state's demographics. Of the Survey Three participants, 57% were extension agents, 23% were WIC service providers, and 20% were Public Health service providers.

Surveys One and Two

Table 1 presents the general folic acid awareness, knowledge, behaviors, and barriers among survey participants of service providers. Survey One data revealed that 315 (74.8%) of participants were aware of folic acid. On Survey Two, 75.8% of participants indicated they were aware of folic acid. The difference in folic acid awareness among survey participants was not significant (p-value >.05). On Survey One, approximately 52.7% knew that folic acid was a vitamin, 1.9% were able to correctly identify five sources of folic acid or folate, and approximately 69.4% knew the recommendation for women to get folic acid to prevent birth defects. Of the Survey Two participants, 45.4% knew how much folic acid was recommended, and 46.1% knew when it should be taken. Differences in folic acid knowledge among participants were significant at the .05 level for responses to all five questions used to measure folic acid knowledge.

Table 1. Folic acid awareness, knowledge, daily intake behavior, and barriers among survey participants

Variable Category	Survey Question Item	Survey One (n=422)		Survey Two (n=349)		Risk Difference	Z[a]	P-value (2-sided)[b]
		No.	%	No.	%			
Awareness	Is aware of folic acid	315	74.82	263	75.79	0.97	0.31025	0.7564
Knowledge	Could identify folic acid	221	52.74	222	64.91	12.17	3.38535	0.0007*
Knowledge	Could identify five sources of folic acid	8	1.90	38	10.95	9.05	5.26047	0.0000*
Knowledge	Could identity why folic acid is needed	292	69.35	277	79.36	10.01	3.14862	0.0016*
Knowledge	Could identify how much folic acid is needed	113	27.16	157	45.37	18.21	5.23313	0.0000*
Knowledge	Could identify when folic acid is needed	137	32.64	160	46.10	13.64	3.86732	0.0001*
Behavior	Does take folic acid daily	174	41.33	198	58.40	17.07	4.68134	0.0000*
Barrier	Reported no perceived barriers to daily folic-acid intake	129	30.56	164	46.99	16.43	4.67619	0.0000*

Note: [a]Z-approximation test for equality of two independent proportions. [b]An asterisk indicates significance at the 0.05 level.

Table 2. Survey Three frequencies of service provider responses (n=30)

	Yes		No	
Survey Item	No.	%	No.	%
Service provider routinely initiates folic acid and NTD discussion with the majority of first-time clients of childbearing age	12	40.0	18	60.0
Script is available to service provider that includes mention of folic acid or NTDs	7	23.3	23	76.7
Service provider is aware of clients who have had an NTD-affected pregnancy	5	16.7	25	83.3

Table 3. Survey Three frequencies of communication about folic acid and NTDs among service providers (n=30)

Survey Item Response	No. %	
Service provider initiates folic acid and NTD discussion with clients on regular basis		
Almost never	5	16.7
Sometimes	15	50.0
Almost always	4	13.3
I don't know	5	16.7
Clients initiate folic acid and NTD discussion with service provider		
Almost never	21	70.0
Sometimes	3	10.0
Almost always	0	0.0
I don't know	6	20.0

Of the participants, 41.3% (in Survey One) and 58.4% (in Survey Two) reported taking a daily folic acid-containing supplement. On Survey One, 30.6% participants reported no perceived barriers to taking a daily supplement containing folic acid. Of the Survey Two participants, 47.0% reported no perceived barriers to taking folic acid. The differences in folic acid behaviors and barriers were significant at the .05 level.

Tables 2 and 3 present the service providers' perceptions of folic acid communication interaction with clients. Of the participants, 23.3% indicated that their agency provides a script to follow that mentions folic acid, when interacting with clients. The majority of participants (60%) reported that they do not routinely initiate folic acid and NTD discussions with women of childbearing age, during first-time appointments, and 50% report that they "sometimes" initiate folic acid and NTD discussion with clients on a regular basis. In contrast, 70% of the participants perceive that clients "almost never" initiate folic acid and NTD discussions with service providers. Of the participants, 16.7% are aware of clients who have had an NTD-affected pregnancy.

Discussion

In their review of worldwide folic acid campaigns, Rofail et al. (2011) identified factors that affect the success or failure of folic acid education campaigns as incomplete outreach, prior awareness and knowledge, closeness to pregnancy, demographic and other personal characteristics. As Rofail et al. (2011) pointed out, the identification of effective and ineffective factors can help identify target audiences often missed in campaigns, and can be used to guide the design and modification of effective health campaign strategies.

Preventative Innovation

Diffusion is a social change model with strong orientations toward development of improved public health. According to Rogers (2003), a *preventative innovation* is a new idea that an individual adopts now in order to lower the probability of some unwanted future event (p. 234). The *Ready or Not* campaign is an example of a preventative innovation. Sponsored by the CDC and implemented by its partners, the *Ready or Not* campaign addressed the scientific relationship between folic acid levels and the risk of NTD development in fetuses (Hammond et al., 2000, p. 4) in an effort to decrease NTDs across the nation. Birth defects are the leading cause of infant mortality and contribute substantially to morbidity and disability in the United States (Committee on Genetics, 1999, p. 325; Bohn, 2004, p. 2). Designed to launch a process to improve public health through folic acid consumption, the *Ready or Not* campaign emphasized folic acid's potential to prevent birth defects. Females of childbearing age were encouraged to consume 400 mcg of folic acid every day to reduce the risk of having an NTD-affected pregnancy.

The unwanted event that is avoided by adopting a preventative innovation is difficult to perceive because it is a nonevent, the absence of something that otherwise might have happened (Rogers, 2003, p. 234). The delayed reward of being prepared for future conception, through timely and adequate folic acid accumulation, is difficult for many individuals to perceive and comprehend. Research findings demonstrate that if women have an adequate accumulation of folic acid in their bodies, starting at least a month before conception, sufficient levels of folic acid can prevent up to 70% of the potential brain and spinal birth defects during fetal development (Hammond et al., 2000, p. 1; CDC, 1992; CDC, 1999a).

As a preventive innovation, the folic acid task force conducted a statewide campaign to educate women of childbearing age about the relationship between timely and adequate folic acid and NTDs. Modeled after the *Ready or Not* campaign, the statewide coalition utilized a concerted effort to emphasize folic acid's potential to prevent birth defects. Task force volunteers distributed promotional materials and used advertising venues to promote the USPHS recommendation. The statewide campaign incorporated a consistent message to effectively encourage women of childbearing age to consume 400 mcg of folic acid every day, in order to reduce the risk of having an NTD-affected pregnancy that they may never experience.

Campaign Objective One stated: Following the intervention, folic acid awareness among female participants will increase to at least 50%. Folic acid awareness for Survey One (74.8%) and Survey Two (75.8%) exceeded the campaign's first objective. Although the change was not significant, it did reflect a small increase (1.0%).

Increases in folic acid knowledge among participants were noted following Survey Two, and the findings were significant. Five questions were used to analyze folic acid knowledge. Objective Two stated: Following the intervention, folic acid knowledge among female participants will increase to at least 50%. Two folic acid knowledge measures exceeded Objective Two. Approximately 64.9% knew that folic acid was a vitamin and 79.4% knew the recommendation for women to get folic acid to prevent birth defects. Although the differences in folic acid knowledge from Survey One to Survey Two were all significant, only two measures exceeded the campaign's second objective.

Campaign Objective Three stated: Following the intervention, self-reported folic acid intake through supplementation among female participants will be greater than 25%. In the present study, following the intervention, 58.4% of the surveyed females reported taking a folic acid supplement every day. The campaign's third objective was measureable and achieved. One explanation for this increase in vitamin consumption may be the reported reduction in the number of females perceiving barriers to vitamin intake.

Following the intervention, 47% of the Survey Two participants perceived no barriers to daily vitamin intake.

Additionally, service provider feedback was gathered in order to explore gaps in folic acid discussions between providers and clients, and to contribute to the development of folic acid and NTD communication. Objective Four stated: Following the intervention and data analysis, educator feedback will help determine gaps in folic-acid related discussions between service providers and clients, and contribute to the development of best practices for folic-acid and NTD communication. Survey Three was designed to explore folic-acid and NTD discussions between service providers and clients, from the perspective of service providers.

Data revealed that a greater number of service providers (60%) do not routinely initiate folic acid and NTD discussion with the majority of first-time clients of childbearing age. Of the service providers, 23.3% indicated that their agency provides a script that mentions folic acid, which can be used to guide communication between service providers and clients. Of the participants, 13.3% indicated that they almost always initiate folic acid and NTD discussion with clients on regular basis, while the majority (50%) will sometimes bring up the topic. Of the responding survey providers, 70% indicated that clients almost never initiate discussions about folic acid and NTDs.

Key to this project was the statewide involvement of volunteer project collaborators, the leveraging of agency funds, and support from commercial vendors and pharmacists. Without the support of so many individuals, commodity groups, and retail establishments, the magnitude of this campaign would not have been possible. Getting the "folic acid every day" message to women of childbearing age remains vital to reducing the number of NTD-affected pregnancies.

Through this project, we were able to recognize an area of opportunity for folic acid education and intervention. As a result of their interactions with women of childbearing age, extension educators, Public Health staff, and WIC nutritionists are a valuable resource for educating women of childbearing age about the need for folic acid and NTD-risk reduction.

The results of this study offer some practical suggestions for service providers communicating to women of childbearing age about the importance of timely and adequate consumption of folic acid every day. For example, implementing a folic acid discussion protocol with women of childbearing age could be instrumental in helping to prevent NTDs among women who are unaware of the relationship between consumption of the vitamin and the potential birth defects. In addition, promotional materials including posters and brochures can be placed in service providers' offices as ongoing reminders of the role folic acid plays in preventing birth defects.

Limitations and Future Research

The implementation of the folic acid study experienced a limitation related to data gathering during Survey Period Two. During the spring of 2009, the state experienced record flooding, which impacted both the survey administrators and survey respondents. Several survey administers were unable to administer additional surveys during Survey Period Two. For example, universities were closed, and survey administrators and respondents were displaced. As a result, the total number of completed surveys for data set two (Survey Two) was lower than originally anticipated.

Survey design was limited in length, which presented another limitation to the folic acid study. In order to maintain the one-page survey length suggested by the coalition members, questions were omitted from the surveys. The collection of additional demographic information from survey participants may have been relevant to the folic acid study analysis. For example, the present survey did not gather responses related to socioeconomic factors of education or income, and these attributes may have influenced an individual's responsiveness to the folic acid campaign. The *Ready or Not* campaign was investigated for its role modeling potential, and it was not compared to other folic acid campaigns. The *Ready or Not* campaign and the current study's campaign were evaluated on the basis of campaign objective achievement.

The application and conceptual framework of developing best practices for folic acid communication among service providers can be advanced further by overcoming limitations to the present study. Although change agents typically do not concentrate their efforts on their most disadvantaged clients (Rogers, 2003, p.383), multiple change agents specifically connected to disadvantaged and hard-to-reach publics were selected as information service providers for this study. During face-to-face communication/appointments with clients, information service providers may have an opportunity to explain in greater detail the USPHS recommendation.

The survey sample for Survey Three was small (n=30), and most of the participants were extension agents. Additionally, the service provider feedback was gathered at the conclusion of the intervention. Therefore, future research could include pre- and post-surveys with service providers designed to assess the application of best practice strategies during client visits.

Service providers' perceptions of folic acid communication during client visits were included; however, client perceptions of folic acid communication were not included. A future study could investigate how service providers communicate with clients about folic acid, and how clients respond to the messages they receive. Survey responses from clients and information service providers could be correlated to reveal folic acideducation gaps that exist from an interpersonal communication perspective. In addition, a future study could include a survey that includes feedback from clients of service providers about folic acid and NTD discussions during office visits.

Conclusion

The results of this study offer some practical suggestions for service providers communicating with women of childbearing age about the importance of timely and adequate consumption of folic acid. This program provided readily-adaptable, novel ideas for public health educators, including bathroom stall ads, coupons, recipe cards, marriage congratulations cards, oral contraceptive packet auxiliary labels and other communication tools designed to promote the folic acid message. Reaching women of childbearing age with the folic acid message is facilitated by the concerted, ongoing efforts of health education personnel working at the individual level and in community-based partnerships. The lessons learned from this program have utility in shaping future public health campaigns coordinated by nutrition and health educators who strive to heighten folic acid awareness, knowledge, and behavior among women of childbearing age.

References

Bentley, J. R., Ferrini, R. L., and Hill, L. L. (1999). Folic acid fortification of grain projects in the U.S. to prevent neural tube defects. *American Journal of Preventative Medicine,16*(3); 264-267.

Berger, J. (2005). Perceived consequences of adopting the Internet into adult literacy and basic education classrooms. *Adult Basic Education, 15,* 103-121.

Bohn, T. (2004). Summary Report 1995. North Dakota Birth Defects Monitoring System. Retrieved December 14, 2009 from http://www.ndhealth.gov/CSHS/docs/birth-defects-report.pdf.

Centers for Disease Control and Prevention. (1992). Recommendations for the use of folic acid to reduce the number of cases of spina bifida and other neural tube defects. *Morbidity and Mortality Weekly Report, 41*(No.RR-14):1-7.

Centers for Disease Control and Prevention. (1999a). Annex A fact sheets for candidate diseases for elimination or eradication. *Morbidity and Mortality Weekly Report, 48*(SU91); 154-203.

Centers for Disease Control and Prevention. (1999b). Knowledge and use of folic acid by women of childbearing age – United States, 1995 and 1998. *Morbidity and Mortality Weekly Report, 48*(16); 325-327.

Centers for Disease Control and Prevention. (2001). Are women with recent live births aware of the benefits of folic acid? *Morbidity and Mortality Weekly Report, 50*(RR06); 3-14.

Centers for Disease Control and Prevention. (2004). Spina bifida and anencephaly before and after folic acid mandate – United States, 1995-1996 and 1999-2000. *Morbidity and Mortality Weekly Report, 53*(17); 362-365.

Committee on Genetics. (1999). Folic acid for the prevention of neural tube defects. *Pediatrics, Vol. 104*(2,); 325-327.

Freimuth, V. S. (1995). Mass media strategies and channels: A review of the use of media in breast and cervical cancers screening programs. *Wellness Perspectives, 11*(2); 79-106.

Hammond, S. L., Squires, L., and Treiman K. (2000). Task 927650: Formative research for folic acid and birth defects prevention. Centers for Disease Control and Prevention. Retrieved from http://www.cdc.gov/DHDSP/ cdcynergy_training/Content/activeinformation/resources/FA_Eval_Plan.pdf

Haider, M., and Kreps, G. (2004). Forty years of diffusion of innovations: Utility and value Inpublic health, *Journal of Health Communication*, 9: 3-11. Doi. 10.1080/10810730490271430.

Heath, R. (2006). Best practices in crisis communication: Evolution of practice through research. *Journal of Applied Communication Research, 34,* 245-248.

Hoover, J. R., Martin, P. A., Litchfield, R. E., (2009, February). Evaluation of a new nutrition education curriculum and factors influencing its implementation. *Journal of Extension, 47*(1); IFEA4. Retrieved March 9, 2010 from http://www.joe.org/joe/2009february/a4.php.

Mason, J. B. (2009). Folate, cancer risk, and the Greek god, Proteus: a tale of two chameleons. *Nutrition Reviews, 67*(4); 206-212.

North Dakota Public Health. (2009). Family Planning. Retrieved December 14, 2009 from http://www.cityoffargo.com/Residential/CityServices/Healthservices/FamilyPlanning/.

Oakley, Jr. G. P. (2007). When will we eliminate folic acid-preventable spina bifida? *Epidemiology, 18*(3); 367-368.

Radimer, K., Bindewald, B., Hughes, J., Ervin, B., Swanson, C., and Picciano, M. F. (2004). Dietary supplement use by US adults: Data from the National Health and Nutrition Examination Survey, 1999-2000. *American Journal of Epidemiology, 160*(4); 339-349.

Rofail, D., Colligs, A., Abetz, L., Lindemann, M., and Maguire, L. (2011). Factors contributing the success of folic acid public health campaigns. *Journal of Public Health* first published online July 3, 2011 doi: 10.1093/pubmed/fdr048.

Rogers, E. (2003). *Diffusion of Innovations.* (5th ed.) New York, NY: The Free Press.

Rogers, E. (2004). A prospective and retrospective look at the diffusion model. *Journal or Health Communication, 9,* 13-19.

Seeger, M. W. (2006). Best practices in crisis communication: An expert panel process. *Journal of Applied Communication Research, 34,* 232-244.

Sellnow, T. L., Ulmer, R. R., Seeger, M. W., and Littlefield, R. S. (2009). *Effective risk communication: A message-centered approach.* New York, NY: Springer.

Steinhaus, J., Brunt, A., Pankow, D., Garden-Robinson, J., and Terbizan, D. (2009, August). Who attends the extension family nutrition program in a rural state, and what are the preferences of its diverse clientele? *Journal of Extension, 47*(4); 4RIB3. Retrieved March 9, 2010 fromhttp://www.joe.org/joe/2009august/rb3.php.

Women Infants and Children. (2009). WIC: The special supplemental nutrition program for women, infants, and children. Retrieved December 14, 2009 from http://www.fns.usda.gov/wic/WIC-Fact-Sheet.pdf.

U.S. Preventive Services Task Force (2009). Folic acid for the prevention of neural tube defects: U.S. Preventive Services Task Force recommendation statement. *Annals of Internal Medicine, 2009, 150:*626-631.

In: Folic Acid
Editors: Mária Szabó and Eve Varga ISBN: 978-1-62100-867-5

Chapter VI

Folic Acid and Prostate Cancer

Oluwakemi Obajimi*
University of Medicine and Dentistry of New Jersey,
Department of Medicine, 401 Haddon Avenue, Camden, NJ, US

Abstract

Increasing evidence continues to indicate that dietary nutrients can significantly influence the incidence of many cancer types. One dietary component that has been implicated as a crucial factor in carcinogenesis is folate. Folate is a water-soluble member of the vitamin B group that plays a key role in DNA methylation, synthesis, and repair. The synthetic form of folate is folic acid, and this form is more biologically available than the natural folate form. While several epidemiological studies suggest that higher folate intake corresponds with decreased risk of many human malignancies, data showing the relationship between folate intake and the risk of prostate cancer are limited and inconsistent. Importantly, a clear demonstration of the benefits of dietary folate for reducing prostate cancer risk is yet to be established. With recent biotechnological capabilities to genetically engineer crops to have increased availability of important biological nutrients, future clinical studies directed at investigating the correlation between folate and chemoprevention of prostate cancer will be challenging but important, coming with the promise to yield high public health benefits.

* Email: kemobaj@yahoo.co.uk.

Introduction

Prostate cancer (PCa) is the most commonly diagnosed cancer in males in economically developed countries [1]. It is one of four cancer forms with rates found to be two- to five- times greater in developed countries than in developing countries [1]. The reason for this disparity is attributed to differences in risk factors, diagnostic practices and the availability of treatment facilities and measures. Prostate cancer is the sixth leading cause of cancer death in males worldwide [1], with an estimated 240,890 new cases and 33,720 deaths to occur in the United States in 2011 [2]. Due to the global prevalence of prostate cancer, the prevention of the disease is an active area of research. The established risk factors for prostate cancer are age, race/ethnicity and family history. These factors can not be modified. Therefore, it is important to examine modifiable measures such as lifestyle and dietary nutrition, with the possibility to lessen the risk of prostate cancer.

Folate is an essential dietary nutrient required for one-carbon metabolic reactions including the synthesis of purine and pyrimidine and also in the conversion of the amino acid, methionine, to *S*-adenosylmethionine (SAM) [3, 4]. Importantly, SAM is a biomolecule that is primarily responsible for the methylation of DNA. Hence, folate deficiency, which can be caused by alcoholism, or the inadequate intake of folate may result in reduced bioavailability of methyl groups for DNA methylation. Essentially, depletion of the precursors required for DNA synthesis and/or repair and leads to the development of cancer [4]. Notably, in prostate tumors, hypomethylation as well as hypermethylation of DNA have been reported [5-9]. DNA hypermethylation of CpG-rich promoter regions is a mechanism known to be involved in the inactivation of tumor suppressors and other genes in the prostate [9, 10]. While DNA hypermethylation acts by changing the expression of selected genes, hypomethylation may promote transcription and recombination throughout the genome by its effect on the structure of the chromatin [8-10].

Although folic acid is the synthetic form of folate that occurs in the oxidized state and contains only one conjugated glutamate residue, natural folates exists as polyglutamates that are hydrolyzed to monoglutamates in the small intestine and then polyglutamylated in peripheral cells [11]. Folate occurs naturally in a variety of foods including broccoli, asparagus, dark-green leafy vegetables, romaine lettuce, liver, whole grain products, wheat germ, chick peas and black-eyed peas. Biological reactions requiring folate are influenced by other essential nutrients including vitamins B-6 and B-12, which act as cofactors [12].

To date, epidemiological studies have linked different cancer types to the folate status. These include colorectal cancer [13, 14], breast cancer [15, 16], ovarian cancer [17], cervical cancer [13], lung cancer [13], gastric cancer [18], pancreatic cancer [19] and esophageal squamous cell carcinoma [20]. In prostate cancer however, there is limited yet conflicting evidence regarding whether high serum levels or increased dietary intake of folate correlates with the reduced risk of developing prostate cancer [21-25]. This brief chapter summarizes some of the important studies that have examined dietary folate intake or circulating levels of folate in prostate cancer patients and defines the current state of knowledge regarding the relationship between folate bioavailability and the incidence and/or progression of prostate cancer.

The Relationship between Dietary Intake of Folate and Prostate Cancer

While some epidemiological studies show evidence that dietary nutrients such as folate and its coenzymes may diminish the risk of prostate cancer and its progression ([26, 27]), others demonstrate that foods such as fat and meat (a major source of vitamin B12), may increase risk [28, 29]. Adequate dietary folate intake, together with the sufficient supply of folate coenzymes, is important for cell division due to the essential role played by folate and its coenzymes in DNA synthesis, methylation and repair. In addition, the rate of serum folate loss via urine, feces, malabsorption and/or folate breakdown influences the amount biologically available for the maintenance of normal cellular metabolism. The two primary mechanisms linking low folate status to carcinogenesis are (a) that inadequate folate may result in reduced levels of SAM leading to DNA hypomethylation thereby promoting cancer growth; and (b) that folate deficiency negatively affects uracil incorporation into DNA thus stressing DNA repair and causing increased DNA strand breaks and chromosomal instability [30].

Serum folate status resulting from inadequate dietary intake has long been postulated to be related to the development and progression of cancer, in general [31]. The role of folate in carcinogenesis pertains to its key function in maintaining the DNA structure, stability and transcriptional control [10, 30]. The occurrence of both hypomethylated and hypermethylated forms of DNA in prostate cancer [5-9] indicates that folate plays a critical role in the pathogenesis of the disease. However, data from several studies regarding the relationship between folate intake and prostate cancer have been inconsistent (Table 1).

Table 1. Summary of studies showing the relationship between dietary folate intake and the risk of prostate cancer

Variables	Pelucchi et al. [24]	Weinstein et al. [26]	Vlajinac et al. [25]	Stevens et al. [27]	Shannon et al. [34]
Study type	Case-Control	Case-Control	Case-Control	Case-Control	Case-Control
[Folate] (μg/d)	196 - 316	234 - 443	69.5 - 264.5	<204 - ≥347	121.2 - 1761.4
Age (years)	46 - 74	50 - 69	~ 70	50 - 74	46 - 86
PCa cases (n)	1,294	1,270	101	5,158	140
Controls (n)	1,451	25,841	202	60,678	480
Total subjects (N)	2,745	27,111	303	65,836	620
Dietary folate relationship with PCa risk	Yes	No	No	Somewhat	Yes
Study duration	1991 - 2002	1985 - 2002	1990 - 1994	1992 - 2001	2001 - 2006
Country	Italy	Finland	Yugoslavia	USA	USA
Other dietary nutrients e.g. Vitamin B6/12	D	D	D	D	D
Alcohol/Smoking	D/D	D/D	ND/ND	D/ND	D/D

D, denotes determined factors; ND, not determined factors and PCa, prostate cancer. These factors were adjusted for in the final analysis.

Data collected between 1985 and 2002 during epidemiological studies of dietary factors of one-carbon metabolic reactions, in a total of 27,111 enrolled Finnish male smokers (1,270 cases; 25,841 controls), aged 50-59 years, reported no protective role for dietary folate intake (234 – 443 μg/day) against the risk of prostate cancer regardless of alcohol consumption [26]. Notably, previous studies have demonstrated that alcohol consumption interferes with folate absorption, metabolism and excretion [32, 33]. In a smaller case-controlled study conducted in Yugoslavia from 1990 to 1994 in 303 men (101 cases; 202 controls) with a mean age of ~70 years, there was no association found between increased dietary folate intake (69.5 – 264.5 μg/day) and the risk of prostate cancer [25]. In the United States, data collected from another epidemiological study over 9 years (1992-2001) in a large cohort of 65,836 subjects (5,158 cases; 60,678 controls), ages 50 – 74 years, showed no relationship between higher dietary folate intake (<204 – ≥347 μg/day) and the incidence of prostate cancer, independent of alcohol consumption [27]. In men with advanced-stage prostate cancer however, higher dietary folate intake marginally lowered prostate cancer risk in prostate specific antigen (PSA)-screened men. Although, this study was statistically limited by the low number of advanced cases (n = 278), results suggest that folate may play a protective role in prostate cancer progression [27].

Interestingly, in an Italian population of high alcohol-consuming men of ages 46 to 74 years, a case-controlled study between 1991 and 2002 of 2,745 enrolled subjects (1,294 cases; 1,451 controls) indicated that dietary intake of folate (196 – 316 μg/day) protected against the risk of prostate cancer [24]. This report further suggested that high intake of alcohol increases bodily requirement for folate and this results in alcohol-folate metabolic interactions that reduce prostate cancer risk [24]. The study showed that the combination of high folate intake with low alcohol consumption produces better outcomes in the prevention of prostate cancer by up to 54% in lowering risk [24]. More recently, epidemiological studies were performed in the United States between 2001 and 2006, in men of ages between 46 and 86 years [34]. Data from 140 biopsy-confirmed prostate cancer patients versus 250 negative prostate biopsy controls (men with normal PSA levels: <4 ng/ml) demonstrated an association between increasing dietary folate intake (121.2 – 1,764.4 μg/day) and the reduced risk of high-grade prostate cancer, regardless of alcohol consumption [34]. Comparisons between 140 biopsy-confirmed prostate cancer cases and 230 age-matched clinical controls (men with elevated PSA levels but no cancer upon biopsy) showed that the intake of dietary folate was inversely proportional with prostate cancer risk [34]. In comparison to age-matched clinical controls, alcohol was however linked to a heightened risk of low-grade prostate cancer [34].

Disparities in the different reports outlined above, pertaining to prostate cancer, encompass the complexities of such epidemiological studies (Table 1). To name a few, confounding factors influencing such clinical studies, include the differences in the concentration of folate ingested, age differences, the existence of other disease conditions, the stage of prostate cancer of individual subjects, racial differences, smoking habits, amount and frequency of alcohol consumption, family history of prostate cancer, the interactions that may occur metabolically between the amount of folate ingested and other nutrients, drug-folate interactions and the accuracy of the answers to the questions on the questionnaires. These and other factors, significantly limit the comparisons and conclusions that can be made between these studies (Table 1). Nonetheless, due to individual genetic differences causing variations in folate absorption, increasing dietary intake of folate does not automatically translate into higher serum concentrations biologically available for folate-requiring metabolic reactions.

The Relationship between Circulating Levels of Folate and Prostate Cancer

In this chapter, we examine results from studies of dietary intake of folate separately from those assessing plasma or serum folate levels because the results are not directly comparable (Table 1 vs. Table 2). Weinstein et al. [21] found no relationship between high serum folate (range studied: <6.87 – >10.79 nM) and the risk of prostate cancer in Finnish subjects (232 cases; 464 controls), ages 50 – 69 years, recruited between 1985 and 1988. In agreement, Hultdin et al. [23] reported no protective role for higher serum folate concentrations (range studied: 3.5 – 14.7 nM) against prostate cancer risk in Swedish patients (254 cases; 514 controls), ages 53 – 63 years, enrolled between 1985 and 2001. In fact, they reported that high serum folate levels may play a role in the promotion of prostate cancer development

[23]. In further support, a case-controlled study performed in Australia between 1990 and 2004 by Beilby et al. [35], in men aged 62 – 77 years, showed no link between serum folate levels (range studied: 3.4 – 102.2 x 10^{-3} nM) and the development of prostate cancer (cases 96; controls 225). Another case-control study (1,461 cases; 1,507 controls) of prostate cancer risk conducted in the United Kingdom between 2001 and 2009, detecting prostate cancer by PSA testing in men, found no association between serum folate concentrations (range studied: <10.8 – >26.2 nM) and risk in men (ages 50-69 years) with localized prostate cancer [36]. This same study found a link between circulating (serum) folate and increased risk of prostate cancer in cohort studies based on clinically detected cases of the disease [36]

.

Table 2. Summary of studies showing the relationship between circulating serum/plasma folate and the risk of prostate cancer

Variables	Weinstein et al. [21]	Hultdin et al. [23]	Beilby et al. [35]	Collin et al. [36]	Rossi et al. [37]	Figueiredo et al. [38]	Tomaszewski et al. [39]	Collin et al. [40]
Study type	Case–Control	Case–Control	Case–Control	Case–Control	Cohort	Placebo-controlled randomized	Case–Control	Cohort
[Folate]/nM	<6.87 - >10.79	3.5 - 14.7	0.0034 - 0.1022	<10.8 - >26.2	0 - ≥0.0136	0.41 - 1.11	22 - 110.8	0.00084 - 0.00111
Age (years)	50 - 69	53 - 63	62 - 77	50 - 69	45 - 69	48 - 66	40 - ≥70	45 - 70
PCa cases (n)	232	254	96	1,461	n/s	n/s	87	424
Controls (n)	464	514	225	1,507	n/s	n/s	20	n/s
Total subjects (N)	696	768	321	2,968	964	643	107	n/s
Circulating folate relationship with PCa risk	No	Somewhat	No	Somewhat	Yes	Yes	Yes	Yes
Study duration	1985 - 1988	1985 - 2001	1990 - 2004	2001 - 2009	1972 - 2001	1994 - 2006	n/s	2000 - 2008
Country	Finland	Sweden	Australia	UK	Australia	USA	USA	UK
Other dietary nutrients e.g. Vitamin B6/12	D	D	D	D	ND	D	D	D
Alcohol/Smoking	ND/ND	ND/D	ND/D	D/D	D/D	D/ND	ND/ND	D/D

D, denotes determined factors; ND, not determined factors; PCa, prostate cancer and n/s, not specified. These factors were adjusted for in the final analysis. Where required, 441.4 is the molecular weight used to calculate the molar concentration of folate.

In contrast however, epidemiological data collected over ≥20 years follow-up period (1972 - 2001) in 964 men in Australia, aged 45 – 69 years, associated lower serum folate levels (range studied: 0 – ≥0.0136 nM) to increased risk of prostate cancer mortality

[37]. Similarly, a recent double-blind randomized clinical trial conducted in the United States, studying data collected between 1994 and 2006 from 643 men, ages 48 – 66 years, randomly assigned to treatment (placebo with/without aspirin: 316; folic acid with or without aspirin: 327) revealed that the plasma folate concentration (range studied: 0.41 – 1.11 nM) was inversely associated with the risk of prostate cancer [38].

Interestingly, recent results from clinical studies also conducted in the United States demonstrated an increased risk of prostate cancer in men (87 cases; 20 controls), 40 to ≥70 years of age, with higher serum folate levels (range studied: 22 – 110.8 nM) [39]. Another study [40] performed in the United Kingdom between 2000 and 2008, assessing serum folate levels (0.84 – 1.11 x 10^{-3} nM) in 424 patients with localized prostate cancer (ages 45-70), indicated that higher folate levels in the serum may be associated with increased PSA velocity, a factor indicative of rapidly progressing disease, including the occurrence of death [41].

Although most, not all of the studies, as summarized in Table 2, were modeled in such a way that the analysis of circulating folate levels were adjusted for potential confounders such as age, alcohol use, dietary intake of vitamins B6 and B12 and folic acid supplementation, the variations in study design may partly explain the contradictory findings. Importantly, folate metabolism itself involves complexities probably suggesting that folate may play a dual role in cellular metabolism [23, 36-40]; in which lower serum concentrations of folate are associated with increased prostate cancer risk and when present in higher levels, promotes the progression of prostate cancer [42]. In other words, some of the studies discussed here-in [23, 36, 39, 40], present evidence in support of a critical role for higher folate concentrations in the facilitation of prostate cancer aggressiveness.

Pharmacological Depletion of Folate by Antifolate Drugs in Prostate Cancer Prevention

Since folate is an essential nutrient (a vitamin) required for optimal growth, cell division, cell development and general health maintenance throughout life, folic acid fortification of food products was implemented in the United States in the mid-1990s and also in many other countries. Besides cancer [30], folate deficiency has been associated with anemia [43], vascular diseases [44], atherosclerosis [45] and neural tube defects [46]. However, exposure to extra folic acid through fortification may be detrimental to those with vitamin B12 deficiency particularly in elderly populations [43]. Therefore, monitoring serum folate levels in some populations is a public health concern.

Folate metabolism, especially its role in DNA methylation in the process of carcinogenesis, has attracted increasing attention. In prostate cancer, the silencing of certain regulatory genes, including tumor suppressors, triggered by DNA hypermethylation and/or hypomethylation of certain regulatory sequences, appears to be a driving force for the development of the disease [5, 6, 8, 9]. Importantly, the bioavailability of methyl groups is dependent on the folate status, with the 5-methyltetrahydrofolate form supplying the methyl groups for the vitamin B12 coenzyme-catalyzed conversion of homocysteine into methionine. Thereafter, methionine is converted into SAM, a universal biological methylating agent involved in numerous methyltransferase reactions including DNA methylation [3]. Furthermore, the misincorporation of uracil into DNA, a phenomenon causing DNA damage, occurs in prostate cancer [47]. Uracil misincorporation was minimized by folate supplementation in folate-deficient cancer patients [30] by its promotion/restoration of thymidylate synthesis from uracil, thus making folate metabolism even more important to study in prostate carcinogenesis.

Since folate is required for DNA synthesis, methylation and repair, dietary manipulation of this vitamin with antifolates, drugs that cause folate deficiencies, has been considered to be a "double-edged sword" at least in the prevention of colorectal cancer

[48]. This is based on results from epidemiological studies that suggest that folate deficiency may promote the development of colorectal cancer while high folate status may enhance its progression [49, 50]. Importantly, pharmacological folate depletion by classical and non-classical antifolate

drugs such as pemetrexed [51], methotrexate [52] and AG2034 [53-55], act by inhibiting cell division, cell growth and progression of cancer cells. On one hand, the use of antifolate drugs may induce genetic and epigenetic damage to cells thereby causing transformations to cancerous cells in previously non-cancer cells. On the other hand, folate supplementation may inhibit cell transformations at the same time producing highly prolific cells, characteristic of tumor growth [42].

In support of a dual role for folate in carcinogenesis [42], clinical reports show conflicting evidence regarding the link between increasing serum folate levels by dietary supplementation and prostate cancer risk [21, 23, 35-40]. In fact, Hultdin et al. [23] showed that high plasma folate levels together with high vitamin B12 concentrations increase prostate cancer risk. However, recent studies showing that prostate cancer cells, in particular, are highly sensitive to folate depletion which in turn induces genomic instability and alters phenotypic characteristics of prostate cancer cells [56], suggest that treatment strategies utilizing antifolate therapies may be particularly effective against prostate cancer cell proliferation and progression.

Over the past 6 decades, a large number of laboratory studies and clinical trials have been directed at enzymes requiring folate as a cofactor, as targets for chemotherapeutic agents [57-60]. Interest in this area of research has steadily increased and proved fruitful for generating and testing novel etiologic hypotheses and new therapeutic agents for a wide range of cancer types [61]. Moreover, cancer treatment with antifolates has produced promising results and is the subject of several ongoing studies and clinical trials in the USA and Europe [62-68]. Since it is widely recognized that prostate cancer treatment along with the prevention of relapse/tumor resistance to treatment improves the patients' prognosis, a better understanding of folate involvement in the onset and progression of the disease, coupled with fundamental knowledge of the basic metabolic pathways governing the transition from early-stage to late-stage prostate cancer would be an extremely important development, highly beneficial to the effective treatment of the disorder with antifolate drugs.

Discussion

While different clinical trials (Table 1 and Table 2) studying the link between increasing concentrations of folate (dietary or circulating) and prostate cancer have found an association with prostate cancer risk or progression [24, 34, 37, 38], others show no correlation with the incidence or advancement of the disease [21, 26, 35]. For instance, in a combined analysis of epidemiological studies performed in Norway between 1998 and 2005 with observational follow-up periods extended through 2007, data from two randomized, double-blind, placebo-controlled clinical trials studying a total of 6,837 subjects with ischemic heart diseases, of which 165 were prostate cancer patients, Ebbing et al. [69] found no association between folic acid treatment and prostate cancer outcomes.

Although lifestyles such as alcohol consumption and smoking habits have been thought to interfere negatively with folate absorption and metabolism [32, 70, 71], epidemiological studies in prostate cancer patients suggest conflicting and inconsistent effects of these factors on prostate cancer outcomes [24, 26, 27, 34]. In fact, one clinical study [24] observed a higher protective role for dietary folate against the risk of prostate cancer in patients consuming high alcohol levels. While some studies have found that alcohol consumption or smoking habits can influence folate status which in turn demonstrates no effect on the risk of prostate cancer [21], others show alcohol-folate interactions that result in increased risk of low-grade prostate cancer [34]. A plausible explanation for inconsistencies in these trial observations may be in the different measures used to gauge metabolically-active folate concentrations. Some studies relate serum or plasma folate levels to prostate cancer risk, others use the concentration ingested through food or supplements to determine the existing folate–prostate cancer relationship. Importantly, increasing dietary folate intake through supplements or fortified foods, does not automatically translate into higher circulating blood levels. This may be due to individual complexities such as inherent genetic differences that may affect folate absorption, drug interactions, influences of other vitamins or dietary nutrients *in vivo*, habits and life style. It is also important to note that the synthetic folate form (folic acid) found in fortified foods is more easily absorbed than natural folate. However, it needs to be reduced in the liver by dihydrofolate reductase before it can enter into the folate cycle. In addition, non-reduced folic acid from fortified foods circulating in the blood stream may compete with cellular metabolism, transport and regulatory functions of natural folate possibly, influencing the effect of folate on prostate cancer risk or progression [72].

Despite the widespread intake of folate as supplements and/or in fortified foods, the benefits and risks associated with the incidence or progression of prostate cancer have not been rigorously studied in patients. Beyond its general health effects, folate intake in prostate cancer patients has unique implications per individual patient and these are further compounded by its potential interactions with other factors such as the current chemotherapeutic drug(s) that the patient is on, age, ethnicity/race, stage of the disease, diet and/or lifestyle. These potential confounding factors, acting alone in folate metabolism or in combination with others, may influence cancer recurrence, progression or even survival. In fact, clinical evidence suggests that folate supplementation can have anti-prostate cancer benefits before tumor development [24, 34] and in other cases, potentially accelerate tumor growth [36]. Thus, it is prudent that the folate status in prostate cancer patients and survivors is closely monitored during treatment.

Besides the reason that the clinical studies discussed here-in were performed in different countries, perhaps the disparities in the reports are due to differences in baseline serum levels of folate in the subjects. After all, recent studies suggest that European men in general, have lower serum folate levels in comparison to men in the United States [39]. This is probably due to the compulsory folic acid fortification of foods in the United States since the late 1990s. Epidemiological evidence suggesting that increased circulating folate can be beneficial to some [24, 34] and detrimental to others [36, 43], questions whether one concentration of folate intake should be used in all patients in each trial. Since prostate cancer risk certainly varies by age, ethnicity/race and family history, a re-evaluation in the manner and timing of folate intervention is warranted in future clinical trials. The design of studies of dietary intake and circulating levels of folate should be modeled as continuous variables with proper and universal adjustments made for potential confounders such as age, amount of fortified foods ingested, basal plasma folate concentrations, supplement intake, smoking habits, alcohol consumption, stage of prostate cancer, metabolic disorders, sample size, sampling frequency, follow-up period and geographic location..

That the process of prostate cancer development is a slow one further complicates the design of prospective studies. In the determination of circulating folate concentrations, a single serum sampling method instead of multiple serum sampling does not assess long-term prostate cancer risks. In addition, uniformity in reports of baseline levels of risk factors such as PSA, race and family history of the recruited patients will be beneficial in future prostate cancer risk studies. Nonetheless, the epidemiological studies discussed here-in highlight the complexities involved in the design of clinical trials towards the determination of the particular role of folate in the prevention, development and/or progression of prostate cancer.

To date, epidemiological evidence for a folate–prostate cancer relationship is limited and inconsistent. Taken together, the studies reported in this chapter support the suggestion that folate plays a dual role in carcinogenesis [42] and that the timing of folate administration may influence disease progression. While increasing the folate status may prevent the development of prostate cancer, its administration after the occurrence of the disease appears to contribute to its progression.

Conclusion

The identification and development of new cancer-chemopreventive agents, including dietary nutrients, especially those specifically effective against particular cancer types and subtypes, continue to be top priority in cancer research. Even though genetic and environmental factors are known contributors, as yet, the etiology of prostate cancer remains unclear. In actual fact, the reason(s) for conflicting associations of folate supplementation, baseline intake or circulating folate levels with prostate cancer carcinogenesis is unknown.

With increasing food fortification with folate, the relationship between folate intake/circulating folate levels and prostate cancer needs further clarification. Nevertheless, this chapter has indicated some important guidelines for a healthy lifestyle with the aim to reduce prostate cancer risk. With the advent of high throughput biotechnological approaches including genomics, transcriptomics, proteomics and metabolomics, these research tools can be used to increase our knowledge of the genes, proteins or metabolites that are differentially affected by high serum folate and in turn prevent or reduce the risk of prostate cancer. For instance, such studies are needed to define dietary manipulations that can be combined with agents that target molecular pathways that can be modulated in order to reduce or prevent cancer cell proliferation.

It has already been established that the risk factors: ethnicity/race, age and family history, for prostate caner are not modifiable. It is also clear that not all men can benefit equally from increased levels of dietary or circulating folate neither will antifolate drug therapy, as attractive as may be, produce similar beneficial results in all prostate cancer cases. Since individual lifestyles, diet and environmental factors may result in inherent genetic differences which in turn can influence the possible anti-cancer effects of most dietary nutrients, knowledge about inter-individual differences in genes associated with prostate cancer risk and/or prevention will be important in the design of future clinical trials studying the relationship between folate and the risk of prostate cancer. Given that circulating folate levels have been associated with prostate cancer risk in some studies, longer-term follow-up stratified studies such as in different ethnic groups/races and in men of different ages with clinical outcomes such as development, metastases and survival are required in order to establish whether folate truly plays a role in the acceleration or prevention of prostate cancer progression.

Without a doubt, future epidemiological research in the area folate status and prostate cancer risk presents huge challenges to the scientific community at large, but at the same time holds promise for great public health benefits.

References

[1] Jemal A, Bray F, Center MM, Ferlay J, Ward E, Forman D: Global cancer statistics. *CA: A Cancer Journal for Clinicians* 2011, 61(2):69-90.

[2] American-Cancer-Society: Cancer Facts and Figures 2011. In. Atlanta: *American Cancer Society*; 2011: 1-60.

[3] Wagner C: Biochemical role of folate in cellular metabolism. In: *Folate in Health and Disease*. Edited by Bailey LB. New York: Marcel Dekker; 1995: 23-42.

[4] Jones PA, Baylin SB: The fundamental role of epigenetic events in cancer. *Nat. Rev. Genet.* 2002, 3(6):415-428.

[5] Santourlidis S, Florl A, Ackermann R, Wirtz H-C, Schulz WA: High frequency of alterations in DNA methylation in adenocarcinoma of the prostate. *The Prostate* 1999, 39(3):166-174.

[6] Lee WH, Morton RA, Epstein JI, Brooks JD, Campbell PA, Bova GS, Hsieh WS, Isaacs WB, Nelson WG: Cytidine methylation of regulatory sequences near the pi-class glutathione S-transferase gene accompanies human prostatic carcinogenesis. *Proceedings of the National Academy of Sciences* 1994, 91(24):11733-11737.

[7] Jarrard DF, Bova GS, Isaacs WB: DNA methylation, molecular genetic, and linkage studies in prostate cancer. *Prostate Suppl.* 1996, 6:36-44.

[8] Yegnasubramanian S, Haffner MC, Zhang Y, Gurel B, Cornish TC, Wu Z, Irizarry RA, Morgan J, Hicks J, DeWeese TL *et al*: DNA

Hypomethylation Arises Later in Prostate Cancer Progression than CpG Island Hypermethylation and Contributes to Metastatic Tumor Heterogeneity. *Cancer Research* 2008, 68(21):8954-8967.

[9] Yegnasubramanian S, Wu Z, Haffner M, Esopi D, Aryee M, Badrinath R, He T, Morgan J, Carvalho B, Zheng Q *et al*: Chromosome-wide mapping of DNA methylation patterns in normal and malignant prostate cells reveals pervasive methylation of gene-associated and conserved intergenic sequences. *BMC Genomics* 2011, 12(1):313.

[10] Schulz WA: DNA methylation in urological malignancies (review). *International Journal of Oncology* 1998, 13(1):151-167.

[11] Lucock M: Folic Acid: Nutritional Biochemistry, Molecular Biology, and Role in Disease Processes. *Molecular Genetics and Metabolism* 2000, 71(1-2):121-138.

[12] Bailey LB, Gregory JF: Folate Metabolism and Requirements. *The Journal of Nutrition* 1999, 129(4):779-782.

[13] Glynn S, Albanes D: Folate and cancer: a review of the literature. *Nutrition and Cancer* 1994, 22(2):101-119.

[14] Giovannucci E, Stampfer MJ, Colditz GA, Hunter DJ, Fuchs C, Rosner BA, Speizer FE, Willett WC: Multivitamin Use, Folate, and Colon Cancer in Women in the Nurses' Health Study. *Annals of Internal Medicine* 1998, 129(7):517-524.

[15] Shrubsole MJ, Shu XO, Li H-L, Cai H, Yang G, Gao Y-T, Gao J, Zheng W: Dietary B Vitamin and Methionine Intakes and Breast Cancer Risk Among Chinese Women. *American Journal of Epidemiology* 2011, 173(10):1171-1182.

[16] Rohan TE, Jain MG, Howe GR, Miller AB: Dietary Folate Consumption and Breast Cancer Risk. *Journal of the National Cancer Institute* 2000, 92(3):266-269.

[17] Larsson SC, Giovannucci E, Wolk A: Dietary Folate Intake and Incidence of Ovarian Cancer: The Swedish Mammography Cohort. *Journal of the National Cancer Institute* 2004, 96(5):396-402.

[18] Kim Y: Folate and carcinogenesis: evidence, mechanisms, and implications. *J Nutr Biochem* 1999, 10:66 - 88.

[19] Oaks BM, Dodd KW, Meinhold CL, Jiao L, Church TR, Stolzenberg-Solomon RZ: Folate intake, post–folic acid grain fortification, and pancreatic cancer risk in the Prostate, Lung, Colorectal, and Ovarian Cancer Screening Trial. *The American Journal of Clinical Nutrition* 2010, 91(2):449-455.

[20] Lu C, Xie H, Wang F, Shen H, Wang J: Diet folate, DNA methylation and genetic polymorphisms of MTHFR C677T in association with the prognosis of esophageal squamous cell carcinoma. *BMC Cancer* 2011, 11(1):91.

[21] Weinstein SJ, Hartman TJ, Stolzenberg-Solomon R, Pietinen P, Barrett MJ, Taylor PR, Virtamo J, Albanes D: Null Association between Prostate Cancer and Serum Folate, Vitamin B6, Vitamin B12, and Homocysteine. *Cancer Epidemiology Biomarkers and Prevention* 2003, 12(11):1271-1272.

[22] Wagner C, Luka Z: Sarcosine, Folate Metabolism and Prostate Cancer—Is There a Link? *The Journal of urology* 2011, 185(2):385-386.

[23] Hultdin J, Van Guelpen B, Bergh A, Hallmans G, Stattin P: Plasma folate, vitamin B12, and homocysteine and prostate cancer risk: A prospective study. *International Journal of Cancer* 2005, 113(5):819-824.

[24] Pelucchi C, Galeone C, Talamini R, Negri E, Parpinel M, Franceschi S, Montella M, La Vecchia C: Dietary Folate and Risk of Prostate Cancer in Italy. *Cancer Epidemiology Biomarkers and Prevention* 2005, 14(4):944-948.

[25] Vlajinac HD, Marinkovic JM, Ilic MD, Kocev NI: Diet and prostate cancer: a case-control study. *European Journal of Cancer* 1997, 33(1):101-107.

[26] Weinstein SJ, Stolzenberg-Solomon R, Pietinen P, Taylor PR, Virtamo J, Albanes D: Dietary factors of one-carbon metabolism and prostate cancer risk. *The American Journal of Clinical Nutrition* 2006, 84(4):929-935.

[27] Stevens VL, Rodriguez C, Pavluck AL, McCullough ML, Thun MJ, Calle EE: Folate Nutrition and Prostate Cancer Incidence in a Large Cohort of US Men. *American Journal of Epidemiology* 2006, 163(11):989-996.

[28] Kolonel LN: Diet. *Epidemiologic Reviews* 2001, 23(1):72-81.

[29] Park S-Y, Murphy SP, Wilkens LR, Henderson BE, Kolonel LN: Fat and meat intake and prostate cancer risk: The multiethnic cohort study. *International Journal of Cancer* 2007, 121(6):1339-1345.

[30] Blount BC, Mack MM, Wehr CM, MacGregor JT, Hiatt RA, Wang G, Wickramasinghe SN, Everson RB, Ames BN: Folate deficiency causes uracil misincorporation into human DNA and chromosome breakage: Implications for cancer and neuronal damage. *Proceedings of the National Academy of Sciences* 1997, 94(7):3290-3295.

[31] Mason JB, Levesque T: Folate: effects on carcinogenesis and the potential for cancer chemoprevention. *Oncology* 1996, 10(11):1727-1736.

[32] Halsted CH, Villanueva JA, Devlin AM, Chandler CJ: Metabolic Interactions of Alcohol and Folate. *The Journal of Nutrition* 2002, 132(8):2367S-2372S.

[33] Shaw S, Jayatilleke E, Herbert V, Colman N: Cleavage of folates during ethanol metabolism. Role of acetaldehyde/xanthine oxidase-generated superoxide. *Biochem. J.* 1989, 257(1):277-280.

[34] Shannon J, Phoutrides E, Palma A, Farris P, Peters L, Forester A, Tillotson CJ, Garzotto M: Folate intake and prostate cancer risk: a case-control study. *Nutrition and Cancer* 2009, 61(5):617-628.

[35] Beilby J, Ambrosini GL, Rossi E, de Klerk NH, Musk AW: Serum levels of folate, lycopene, [beta]-carotene, retinol and vitamin E and prostate cancer risk. *Eur. J. Clin. Nutr.* 2010, 64(10):1235-1238.

[36] Collin SM, Metcalfe C, Refsum H, Lewis SJ, Zuccolo L, Smith GD, Chen L, Harris R, Davis M, Marsden G *et al*: Circulating Folate, Vitamin B12, Homocysteine, Vitamin B12 Transport Proteins, and Risk of Prostate Cancer: a Case-Control Study, Systematic Review, and Meta-analysis. *Cancer Epidemiology Biomarkers and Prevention* 2010, 19(6):1632-1642.

[37] Rossi E, Hung J, Beilby JP, Knuiman MW, Divitini ML, Bartholomew H: Folate Levels and Cancer Morbidity and Mortality: Prospective Cohort Study from Busselton, Western Australia. *Annals of epidemiology* 2006, 16(3):206-212.

[38] Figueiredo JC, Grau MV, Haile RW, Sandler RS, Summers RW, Bresalier RS, Burke CA, McKeown-Eyssen GE, Baron JA: Folic Acid and Risk of Prostate Cancer: Results From a Randomized Clinical Trial. *Journal of the National Cancer Institute* 2009, 101(6):432-435.

[39] Tomaszewski JJ, Cummings JL, Parwani AV, Dhir R, Mason JB, Nelson JB, Bacich DJ, O'Keefe DS: Increased cancer cell proliferation in prostate cancer patients with high levels of serum folate. *The Prostate* 2011:n/a-n/a.

[40] Collin SM, Metcalfe C, Refsum H, Lewis SJ, Davey Smith G, Cox A, Davis M, Marsden G, Johnston C, Lane JA *et al*: Associations of Folate, Vitamin B12, Homocysteine, and Folate-Pathway Polymorphisms with Prostate-Specific Antigen Velocity in Men with Localized Prostate Cancer. *Cancer Epidemiology Biomarkers and Prevention* 2010, 19(11):2833-2838.

[41] van den Bergh RCN, Roemeling S, Roobol MJ, Wolters T, Schröder FH, Bangma CH: Prostate-Specific Antigen Kinetics in Clinical Decision-Making During Active Surveillance for Early Prostate Cancer--A Review. *European Urology* 2008, 54(3):505-516.

[42] Kim Y: Folate: a magic bullet or a double edged sword for colorectal cancer prevention? *Gut* 2006, 55:1387 - 1389.

[43] Selhub J, Paul L: Folic acid fortification: Why not vitamin B12 also? *BioFactors* 2011:n/a-n/a.

[44] Selhub J, Jacques PF, Wilson PW, Rush D, Rosenberg IH: Vitamin status and intake as primary determinants of homocysteinemia in an elderly population. *Journal of American Medical Association* 1993, 270(22).

[45] McCully KS: Homocysteine, vitamins, and vascular disease prevention. *The American Journal of Clinical Nutrition* 2007, 86(5):1563S-1568S.

[46] Sutton M, Mills JL, Molloy AM, Troendle JF, Brody LC, Conley M, Mc Donnell R, Scott JM, Kirke PN: Maternal folate, vitamin B12 and homocysteine levels in pregnancies affected by congenital malformations other than neural tube defects. *Birth Defects Research Part A: Clinical and Molecular Teratology* 2011:n/a-n/a.

[47] Pulukuri SMK, Knost JA, Estes N, Rao JS: Small Interfering RNA–Directed Knockdown of Uracil DNA Glycosylase Induces Apoptosis and Sensitizes Human Prostate Cancer Cells to Genotoxic Stress. *Molecular Cancer Research* 2009, 7(8):1285-1293.

[48] Kim Y-I: Folate: a magic bullet or a double edged sword for colorectal cancer prevention? *Gut* 2006, 55(10):1387-1389.

[49] Kim Y-I: Folate and colorectal cancer: An evidence-based critical review. *Molecular Nutrition and Food Research* 2007, 51(3):267-292.

[50] Ulrich CM, Potter JD: Folate and Cancer—Timing Is Everything. *JAMA: The Journal of the American Medical Association* 2007, 297(21):2408-2409.

[51] Bischof M, Abdollahi A, Gong P, Stoffregen C, Lipson KE, Debus Jü, Weber KJ, Huber PE: Triple combination of irradiation, chemotherapy (pemetrexed), and VEGFR inhibition (SU5416) in human endothelial and tumor cells. *International journal of radiation oncology, biology, physics* 2004, 60(4):1220-1232.

[52] Elder JS, Gibbons RP: Results of trials of the USA National Prostatic Cancer Project. *Progress in Clinical and Biological Research* 1985, 184A:221-242.

[53] Obajimi O, Melera P: The depletion of cellular ATP by AG2034 mediates cell death or cytostasis in a hypoxanthine-dependent manner in human prostate cancer cells. *Cancer Chemotherapy and Pharmacology* 2008, 62(2):215-226.

[54] Obajimi O, Keen JC, Melera PW: Inhibition of de novo purine synthesis in human prostate cells results in ATP depletion, AMPK activation and induces senescence. *The Prostate* 2009, 69(11):1206-1221.

[55] Obajimi O, Melera PW: ERK Suppression in DU145 Cells Selected for AG2034 Resistance is Associated with Decreased ATP, GARF Inactivation and Increased ERK Signaling. *The Open Drug Resistance Journal* 2011, 1:1-11.

[56] Bistulfi G, VanDette E, Matsui S-I, Smiraglia D: Mild folate deficiency induces genetic and epigenetic instability and phenotype changes in prostate cancer cells. *BMC Biology* 2010, 8(1):6.

[57] Bosson G: Reduced folate carrier: biochemistry and molecular biology of the normal and methotrexate-resistant cell. *British Journal of Biomedical Science* 2003, 60(2):117-129.

[58] Gangjee A, Shi J, Queener S, Barrows L, RL K: Synthesis of 5-methyl-5-deaza nonclassical antifolates as inhibitors of dihydrofolate reductases and as potential antipneumocystis, antitoxoplasma, and antitumor agents. *Journal of Medicinal Chemistry* 1993, 36(22):3437-3443.

[59] Gangjee A, Jain H, Kurup S: Recent advances in classical and non-classical antifolates as antitumor and antiopportunistic infection agents: part I. *Anticancer Agents Med. Chem.* 2007, 7(5):524-542.

[60] Gangjee A, Jain H, Kurup S: Recent advances in classical and non-classical antifolates as antitumor and antiopportunistic infection agents: Part II. *Anticancer Agents Med. Chem.* 2008, 8(2):205-231.

[61] McGuire J: Anticancer antifolates: current status and future directions. *Current Pharmaceutical Design* 2003, 9(31):2593-2613.

[62] Gkiozos I, Charpidou A, Syrigos K: Developments in the Treatment of Non-small Cell Lung Cancer. *Anticancer Research* 2007, 27(4C):2823-2827.

[63] Gish RG, Porta C, Lazar L, Ruff P, Feld R, Croitoru A, Feun L, Jeziorski K, Leighton J, Knox J *et al*: Phase III Randomized Controlled Trial Comparing the Survival of Patients With Unresectable Hepatocellular Carcinoma Treated With Nolatrexed or Doxorubicin. *Journal of Clinical Oncology* 2007, 25(21):3069-3075.

[64] A phase II study of pemetrexed (alimta) as second-line therapy for hormone refractory prostate cancer: Hoosier Oncology Group GU03-67. ClinicalTrials.gov Identifier: NCT00216099.

[65] A phase II trial of oxaliplatin and pemetrexed in hormone refractory prostate cancer. ClinicalTrials.gov Identifier: NCT01338792.

[66] Phase I dose escalation trial of biweekly alimta (with vitamin supplementation) in combination with taxotere in advanced solid tumor patients. ClinicalTrials.gov Identifier: NCT01172028.

[67] A phase 1/2, multicenter, dose-escalation study to determine the safety, efficacy and pharmacokinetics of TH-302 in combination with a) gemcitabine or b) docetaxel or c) pemetrexed in patients with advanced solid tumors. ClinicalTrials.gov Identifier: NCT00743379.

[68] Maintenance treatment for ovarian carcinoma in remission by an antiangiogenic treatment strategy with metronomic/oral chemotherapy (cytophosphan combined with low-dose methotrexate)and COX-2 inhibition (celecoxib). ClinicalTrials.gov Identifier: NCT01175772.

[69] Ebbing M, Bønaa KH, Nygård O, Arnesen E, Ueland PM, Nordrehaug JE, Rasmussen K, Njølstad I, Refsum H, Nilsen DW *et al*: Cancer Incidence and Mortality After Treatment With Folic Acid and Vitamin B12. *JAMA: The Journal of the American Medical Association* 2009, 302(19):2119-2126.

[70] Mannino D, Mulinare J, Ford E, Schwartz J: Tobacco smoke exposure and decreased serum and red blood cell folate levels: data from the Third National Health and Nutrition Examination Survey. *Nicotine Tob. Res.* 2003, 5(3):357-362.

[71] Piyathilake C, Macaluso M, Hine R, Richards E, Krumdieck C: Local and systemic effects of cigarette smoking on folate and vitamin B- 12. *The American Journal of Clinical Nutrition* 1994, 60(4):559-566.

[72] Smith AD, Kim Y-I, Refsum H: Is folic acid good for everyone? *The American Journal of Clinical Nutrition* 2008, 87(3):517-533.

In: Folic Acid
Editors: Mária Szabó and Eve Varga
ISBN: 978-1-62100-867-5

Chapter VII

Photobiological Properties of Folic Acid and its Application

Kazutaka Hirakawa
Department of Basic Engineering (Chemistry),
Faculty of Engineering, Shizuoka University, Johoku 3-5-1,
Naka-ku, Hamamatsu, Shizuoka, Japan

Abstract

Folic acid is an important human nutrient. This compound consists of *p*-aminobenzoyl-L-glutamic acid and pteridine, which absorb ultraviolet A (UVA) light. UVA-irradiation to folic acid results in the decomposition and the formation of unconjugated pteridines through intra-molecular electron transfer and subsequent reactions. The formed pteridines act as strong photosensitizer to damage DNA via electron transfer from guanines, leading to the formation of various oxidized products, including 8-oxo-7,8-dihydro-2'-deoxyguanine, a main indicator of oxidative DNA damage. These findings suggest that photolysis of folic acid may contribute to skin cancer by solar UVA radiation. The conjugation of the pteridine and the aminobenzoyl moiety in folic acid structure may play an important role in the prevention of UVA carcinogesis. On the other hand, fluorescence intensity of folic acid, which scarcely fluoresces, is markedly enhanced by reactive oxygen species through oxidative decomposition. This character can be applied for the fluorometry of hydrogen peroxide and the determination of singlet oxygen quantum yields of various photosensitizers.

1. Introduction

Folic acid, which consists of the base pteridine and *p*-aminobenzoyl-L-glutamic acid (Figure 1), is one of the water-soluble B vitamins essential for human nutrition. The human body requires folic acid to synthesize and to repair DNA. Supplement of folic acid is useful for prevention of cancer [1,2], neural tube defects [3,4], and other disorders [5].

Pteridine moiety of folic acid analogues absorbs the ultraviolet-A (UVA, 320~400 nm), leading to various photochemical reactions from its photoexcited state [6-10]. One of the most important reactions is photo-induced electron transfer. This reaction may contribute to UVA carcinogenesis [11]. Exposure to solar UV radiation is undoubtedly linked to skin carcinogenesis [12]. It is generally recognized that solar UVA carcinogenesis involves a mechanism by which UVA radiation indirectly induces DNA damage through photosensitized reactions mediated by intracellular chromophores [13, 14]. Pteridines, including folic acid and its analogues, might be important endogenous photosensitizers [8,15]. On the other hand, photochemical reaction causes strongly fluorescence enhancement of folic acid analogues [8,9]. The fluorescence enhancement can be induced by photochemical reaction or reactive oxygen species (ROS) [16,17].

This fluorescence enhancement mechanism is similar to that of fluorescence probes to detect ROS and reactive intermediates of peroxide [18], suggesting that folic acids can be applied in the photobiological study concerning photosensitized ROS generation. In this chapter, the photochemical and photobiological properties of folic acid concerning photosensitized DNA damage and their applications in fluorometry of ROS are described.

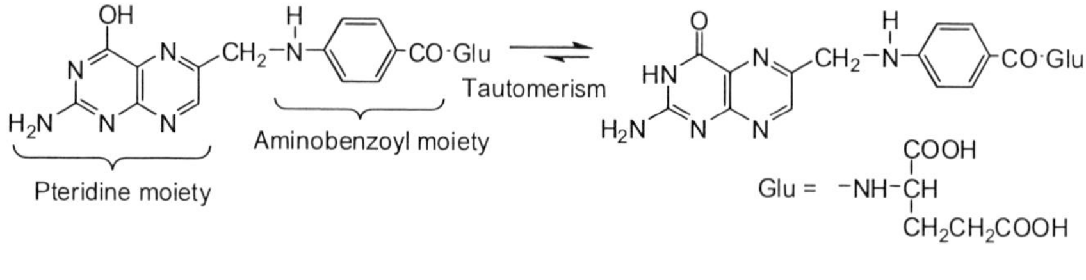

Figure 1. Structure of folic acid.

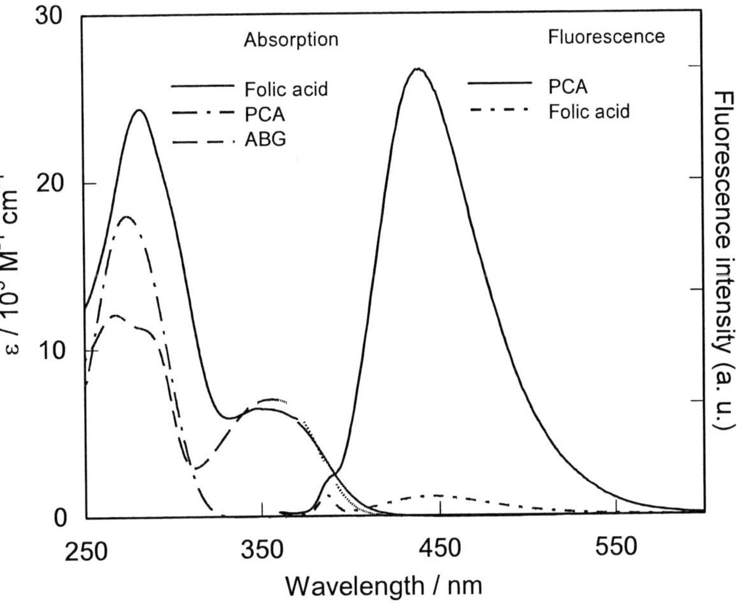

Figure 2. Absorption spectra of folic acid and the related compounds.

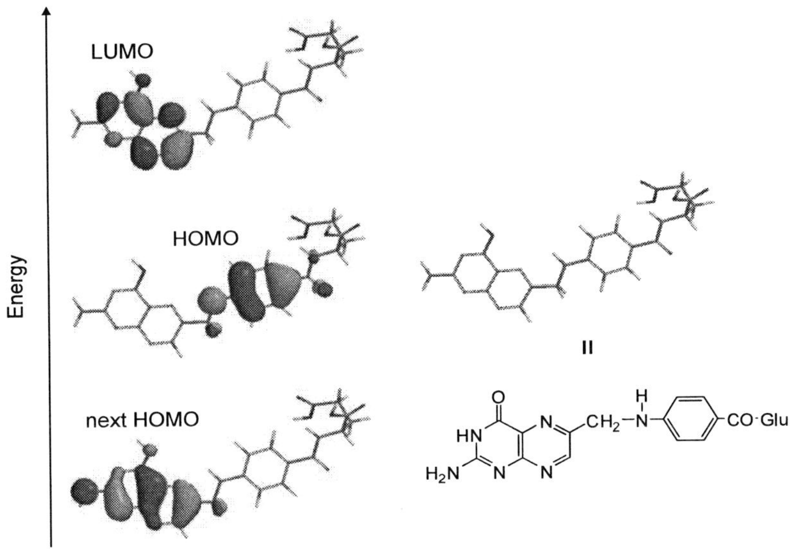

Figure 3. Calculated energy level of folic acid.

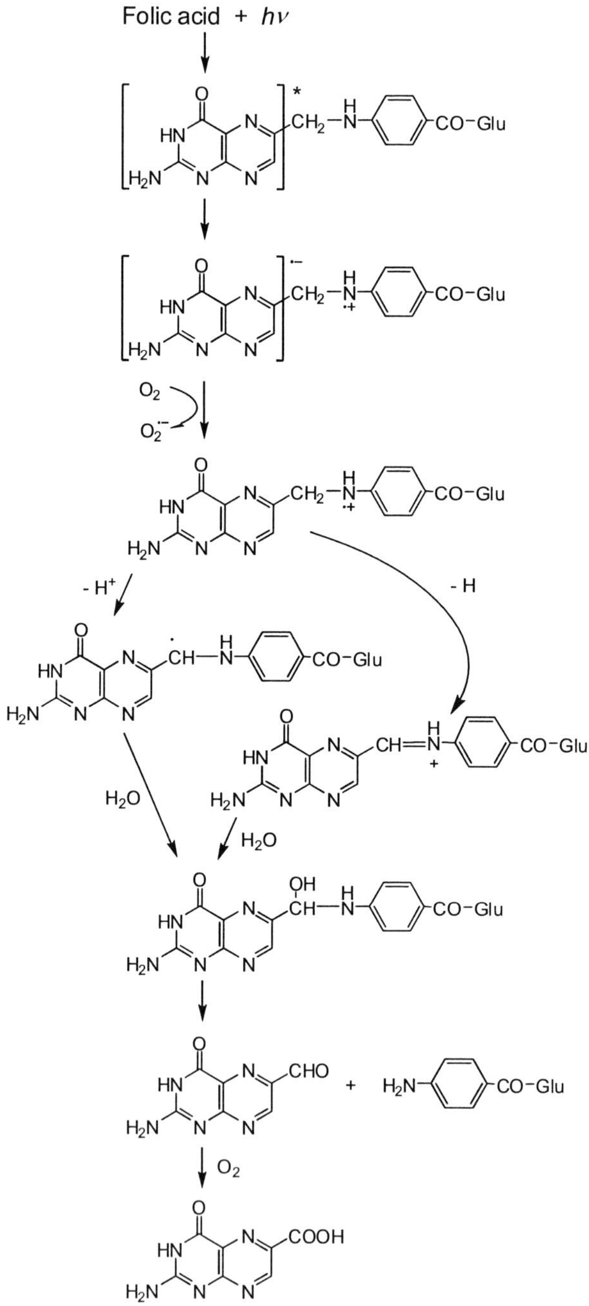

Figure 4. Proposed mechanism of photodecomposition of folic acid.

2. Photochemical Property of Folic Acid

2.1. Direct Photodecomposition of Folic Acid by UVA

Folic acid analogues, conjugated pteridine compounds, consist of the base pteridine and *p*-aminobenzoyl-*L*-glutamic acid. The pteridine moiety absorbs UVA light and emits fluorescence in visible-light region (around 450 nm) (Figure 2) [8]. Fluorescence intensity of the pteridine moiety of folic acid was very weak compared with that of unconjugated pteridines [19].

The reported value of the fluorescence quantum yield (Φ_f) of folic acid is $< 5\times10^{-3}$ [19], whereas the order of those of unconjugated pteridines is $\sim10^{-1}$ [17,19]. The calculated energy levels of the highest-occupied molecular orbital (HOMO), the next HOMO, and the lowest-unoccupied molecular orbital (LUMO) are shown in Figure 3 [16].

This calculation showed that the HOMO is located on the aminobenzoyl moiety of folic acid, suggesting that the fluorescence from the pteridine moiety can be quenched through intra-molecular electron transfer from the aminobenzoyl moiety [8,16].

It has been reported that the free energy change of the electron transfer from the aminobenzoyl moiety to the pteridine moiety is negative (-0.75 eV) [10], supporting the possibility of the photoinduced intra-molecular electron transfer. Indeed, the photoinduced electron transfer from the photoexcited triplet state was demonstrated [10].

When folic acid was previously treated with UVA-irradiation in aqueous solution, the fluorescence intensity increased depending on the extent of UVA light, indicating that UVA light converts folic acid into a stronger fluorescent molecule. The fluorescence spectrum of UVA-irradiated folic acid was quite similar to that of pterin-6-carboxylic acid (PCA). It has been reported that the UVA degradation of folic acid forms PCA and *p*-aminobenzoyl-L-glutamic acid (ABG) [6,7]. Photolysis product of folic acid can be analyzed by high-performance liquid chromatography (HPLC). The generation of PCA was not stoichiometric with the loss of folic acid, suggesting other routes of folic acid degradation and/or the further decomposition of PCA [8]. One of the possibilities is the formation of 6-formylpterine (FPT) [20-22] as an intermediate of PCA from the folic acid decomposition. The following mechanism of PCA generation from photo-excited folic acid can be proposed (Figure 4). The photoexcited state of folic acid is quenched through an intra-molecular electron transfer from the aminobenzoyl moiety to the photo-excited pteridine moiety. The intra-molecular electron transfer rate constant (k_{et}) was roughly estimated to be > 10^9~10^{10} s^{-1} from the relative fluorescence quantum yield of folic acid [8]. Therefore, photo-irradiated folic acid should form radical ion pair, which undergoes hydrolysis and oxidation, leading to the formation of PCA. The above electron transfer from the triplet-excited state of folic acid is also possible [10].

2.2. Photosensitized Decomposition of Folic Acid

Unconjugated pteridines including PCA and FPT can act as photosensitizers to photooxidize organic molecules, such as DNA [8,16]. The formed PCA and FPT sensitize the degradation of folic acid, and this UVA degradation of folic acid is accelerated [9]. Folic acid can be decomposed by photoexcited riboflavin [23], which is also a photosensitizer to induce DNA damage through photoinduced electron transfer [24]. These photoexcited sensitizers should abstract electron from the aminobenzoyl moiety of folic acid, resulting in the similar process in the above-mentioned decomposition (Figure 5).

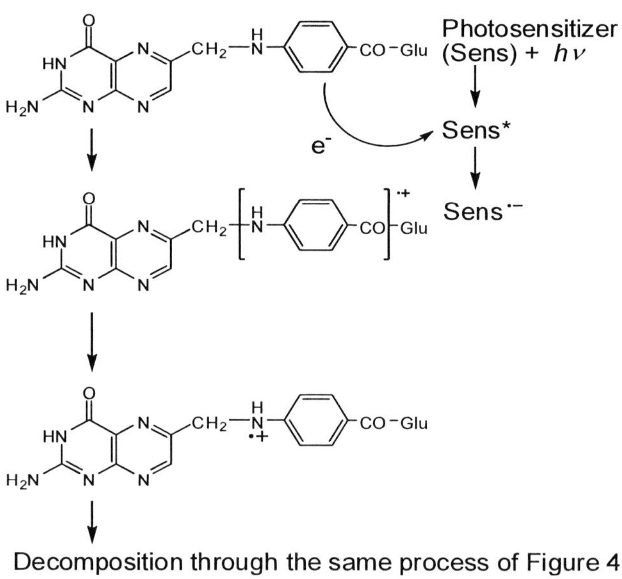

Figure 5. Decomposition of folic acid through photosensitized reaction. The decomposed products of folic acid also act as the photosensitizer.

Recently, it was reported that the singlet excited state of riboflavin mainly decomposes folic acid via electron abstraction, while the contribution of the triplet excited sate to the folic acid decomposition is small [25]. Because riboflavin, a "visible-light photosensitizer", can absorb around 450 nm, the decomposition of folic acid in human skin may be induced by visible-light irradiation as well as UV-irradiation.

2.3. Photodecomposition of a Folic Acid Analogue, Methotrexate

Folic acid analogues may be decomposed by UV or visible-light irradiation. The photochemical stability and the excited state property of pharmaceutical substances should be related to the occurrence of phototoxicity as adverse side effects after drug administration to the patients [26]. Methotrexate (MTX, Figure 6), a folic acid analogue, is a strong inhibitor of dihydrofolate reductase. It has been widely used for chemotherapy for many types of cancer [27]. In addition, MTX has been used in the treatment of psoriasis [28].

MTX absorbs UVA light, and the fluorescence intensity of the pteridine moiety of MTX was very weak (almost no fluorescent) compared with that of unconjugated pteridines similar to folic acid [17].

When MTX was previously treated with UVA irradiation (365 nm), the fluorescence intensity increased depending on the extent of UVA-irradiation, indicating that UVA can convert MTX into a stronger fluorescent molecule [29]. This UVA-induced decomposition of MTX has been studied and reported [29-31]. The photoproducts of MTX decomposition are 2,4-diamino-6-formylpteridine (DFP) and 2,4-diaminopteridine-6-carboxylic acid (DPC). In addition, it was reported that 2,4-diamino-6-hydroxymethylpteridine (DHP) was detected as a decomposed product of MTX [29].

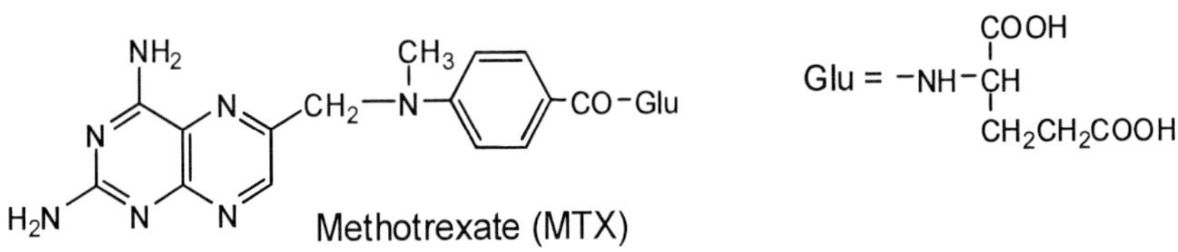

Figure 6. Structure of MTX.

In the HPLC measurement, the peak height of MTX was decreased by photo-irradiation, and the peak of a photolysis product was observed. The retention time and the absorption spectrum of the photolysis product were similar to those of DHP. Furthermore, photoproduct of MTX was analyzed with a mass spectrometer, and the mass spectrum with molecular ion at m/e 192 (M^+) was obtained, confirming the formation of DHP. The mechanism of the MTX degradation by UVA has been proposed as shown in Figure 7.

The photoexcited state of the pteridine moiety of MTX formed by UVA irradiation is quenched through intra-molecular electron transfer. The formed radicals decomposed through hydrolysis, leading to the formation of DHP. Another process of the MTX decomposition leads to the formation of DFP, which may undergo further oxidation into DPC by molecular oxygen.

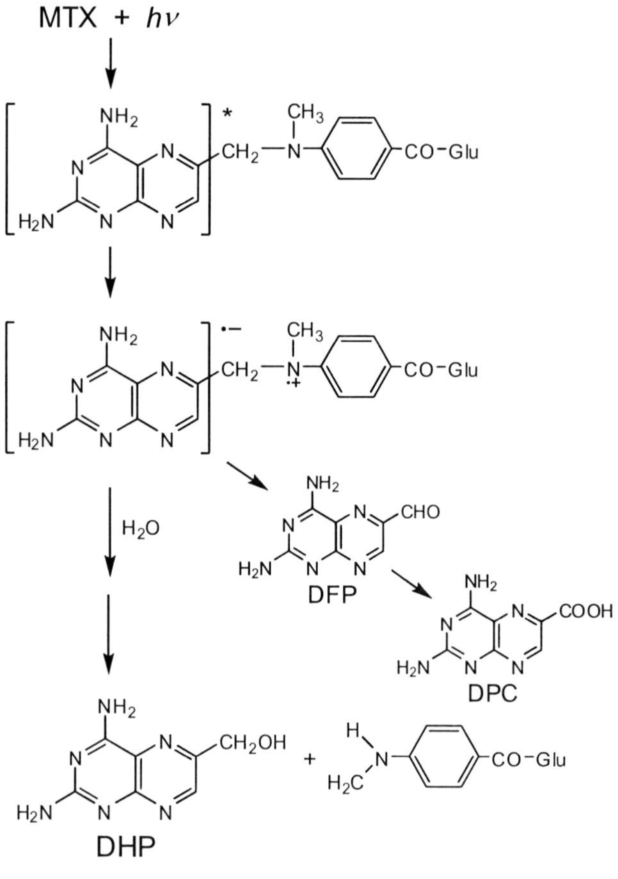

Figure 7. Proposed mechanism of photodecomposition of MTX.

3. Phototoxic Effect of Folic Acid Analogues

3.1. Photocarcinogenesis and UVA-Induced DNA damage

Exposure to solar UV radiation is undoubtedly linked to skin carcinogenesis [12]. It has been well demonstrated in early studies that UVB radiation, which constitutes about 5% of the solar UV radiation that reaches the surface of the earth, directly activates the DNA molecule to generate dipyrimidine photoproducts such as cyclobutane pyrimidine dimers and pyrimidine (6-4) pyrimidone photoadducts, resulting in mutations and carcinogenesis. However, recent studies have provided sufficient evidence that UVA radiation, which accounts for the major portion of the solar UV radiation, is also mutagenic and carcinogenic, although it is unlikely that UVA directly activates DNA bases to produce dipyrimidine photoproducts [32,33]. It is, therefore, generally recognized that solar UVA carcinogenesis involves a mechanism by which UVA radiation indirectly induces DNA damage through photosensitized reactions mediated by intracellular chromophores. Accordingly, a variety of cellular compounds have been considered to be potential endogenous photosensitizers. Folic acid is essential for human nutrition and absorbs UVA region. Therefore, folic acid and its related compounds may act as endogenous UVA photosensitizers. Folic acid is easily decomposed by sunlight and UV light and photodegradation in human skin [34]. UVA-irradiated folic acid generates PCA [6-10]. Therefore, we must consider PCA as photosensitizer, when the photochemical reaction of folic acid is investigated.

3.2. Photosensitized DNA Damage by Folic Acid

It has been demonstrated that UVA irradiation caused DNA damage in the presence of folic acid or PCA [8]. The extent of DNA damage induced by UVA plus PCA was significantly greater than that induced by UVA plus folic acid. The DNA cleavage was observed only when the DNA fragment was treated with piperidine, suggesting that base modification is induced by UVA-irradiated folic acid or PCA. The piperidine treatment can cleave DNA strand at the damaged base. These piperidine-labile products were formed specifically at the underlined G of 5'-GG-3', 5'-GGG-3', and 5'-GGGG-3' sequences by UVA-irradiated folic acid or PCA (Figure 8).

Escherichia coli formamidopyrimidine-DNA glycosylase (Fpg) treatment as well as piperidine treatment demonstrated that photo-excited PCA caused preferential DNA cleavage at consecutive guanine residues in double-stranded DNA. Fpg is known to recognize 8-oxo-7,8-dihydro-2'-deoxyguanosine (8-oxodGuo), as well as 2,6-diamino-4-hydroxy-5-formamidopyrimidine residues [35]. These damaged bases can be removed by Fpg and can be detected by an electrophoresis.

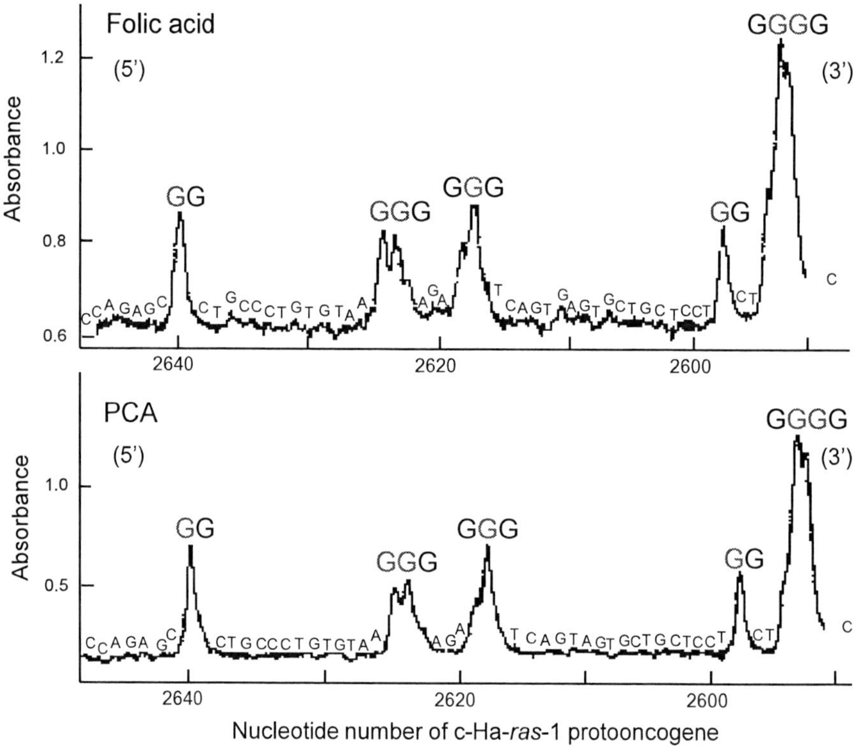

Figure 8. Sequence-specificity of DNA damage by photo-irradiated folic acid and PCA.

These results suggest that photo-excited PCA produces 8-oxodGuo and subsequently piperidine-labile site at consecutive guanine residues in double-stranded DNA. Indeed, the formation of 8-oxodGuo was confirmed with an HPLC. The amount of 8-oxodGuo formation increased depending on concentration of folic acid or PCA. Formation of 8-oxodGuo by folic acid or PCA increased depending on the photo-irradiation dose. The 8-oxodGuo formation by PCA was markedly larger than that by folic acid. No or little DNA damage was induced by UVA in the presence of folic acid within 2 J cm^{-2} (365 nm). The concentration of folic acid decreased, whereas that of PCA generated from folic acid increased, depending on the photo-irradiation dose. The induction period within 2 J cm^{-2} suggests that folic acid itself could cause no or little DNA oxidation, and photoproduct generated from photo-irradiated folic acid, PCA, participates in DNA oxidation. It can be explained by the rapid intra-molecular electron transfer ($k_{et} > 10^9$-10^{10} s^{-1}) leading to the PCA formation preferentially occurs rather than intermolecular reaction of DNA with the photo-excited state of folic acid (the maximum reaction rate constant estimated from the diffusion control limit $\approx 1.8\times10^5$ s^{-1}) [8]. Consequently, DNA damage is due to photoactivation of PCA generated from folic acid rather than folic acid itself.

3.3. The Mechanism of DNA Damage by UVA in the Presence of Folic Acid

The sequence-specificity of DNA damage by photo-excited PCA was quite similar to that induced by type I photosensitizers [11,13,24]. These results suggest that photo-excited PCA oxidizes nucleobase through electron transfer (type I mechanism, Figure 9), leading to the formation of 8-oxodGuo and/or related photoproducts (Figure 10). Electron paramagnetic resonance (EPR) spin destruction method also supported the type I mechanism. EPR signal of 2,2,6,6-tetramethyl-4-piperidone-N-oxyl (4-oxo-TEMPO) radical was clearly observed after photo-irradiation in the presence of PCA [8]. The signal was completely diminished in the presence of guanine. This result can be explained by assuming that 4-oxo-TEMPO radical was diminished by the reaction with guanine cation radical generated through photo-induced electron transfer to photo-excited PCA.

Guanine is most easily oxidized among the four DNA bases, because the oxidation potential of guanine is lower than the other DNA bases [36-38]. Molecular orbital calculations have revealed that stacking of two guanine bases in double-stranded DNA significantly lowers the ionization potential, and electron-loss centers are localized on the consecutive G sequences [39,40]. In our study, it has been confirmed that the amount of 8-oxodGuo formation by photo-excited PCA in double-stranded DNA was larger than that in single-stranded DNA, supporting the DNA damage by this mechanism [11,13,24]. Thus, guanine radical cation formed in DNA is finally localized on consecutive guanine site through charge migration. The decomposition of guanine radical cation might take two competitive pathways: deprotonation followed by reaction with O_2 leading to piperidine-labile product (e.g. imidazolone, oxazolone) [36,41] or hydration leading to 8-oxodGuo [36,41-43], the latter being less efficiently cleaved by hot piperidine treatment [44,45].

Piperidine-labile products can be also formed from 8-oxodGuo through further oxidation [36,46-48]. The relative probability of hydration vs. deprotonation of the radical cation is modulated by the local helical condition and dynamics variations of DNA [45]. PCA anion radical generated through the electron transfer can be converted into PCA through oxidation by molecular oxygen and/or may undergo decomposition.

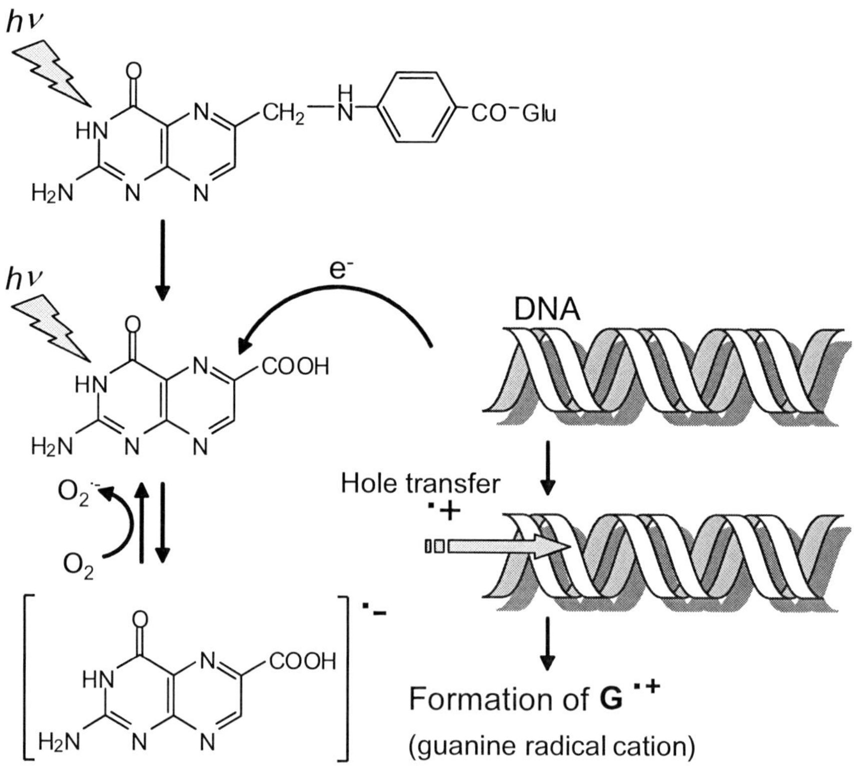

Figure 9. The mechanism of DNA damage by UVA-irradiated folic acid.

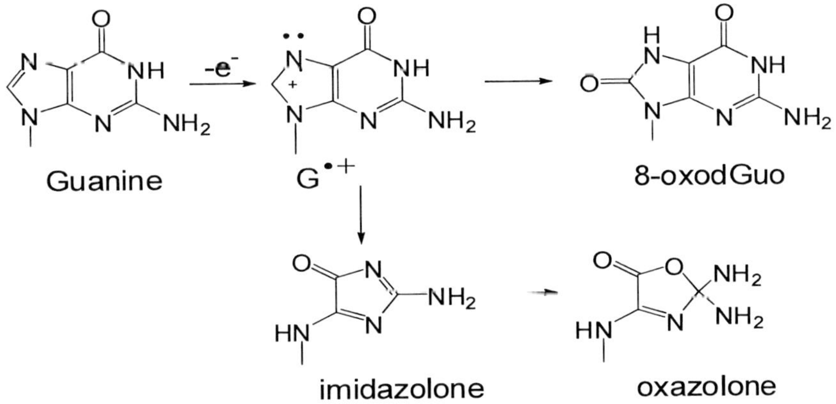

Figure 10. The formation of guanine oxidized products from the guanine radical cation.

3.4. Photobiological Significance of Folic Acid

The formation of 8-oxodGuo causes DNA misreplication may lead to mutation such as G-C → T-A transversion [49,50]. The imidazolone residue formed in DNA may cause G-C → C-G transversion [51,52], due to the formation of stable base pair with G comparable with the Watson-Crick G-C base pair [46,47]. These transversions can explain a part of the mutation induced by UVA radiation as previously reported [32,53]. Photo-irradiated folic acid induces poly-G specific DNA oxidation through photo-induced electron transfer. The reactive species to induce the DNA oxidation is mainly photo-excited PCA, which is generated via photolysis of folic acid. Since folic acid in human skin is easily decomposed by sunlight [34], PCA, an active photosensitizer, may be generated in human skin. Although the pteridine is UVA-photosensitizer, folic acid is an important human nutrition. The connection of the pteridine moiety with the aminobenzoyl moiety plays an important role in the inhibition of DNA damage. This connection may contribute to the prevention of UV carcinogenesis. Therefore, a biological importance in the chemical structure of folic acid is speculated.

3.5. Photosensitized DNA Damage by MTX

Phototoxic effects of MTX have been reported as adverse side effects after administration of MTX to the patients [54-57]. Furthermore, MTX also causes phototoxic effects as adverse side effects of PUVA therapy after administration [55-57]. Since MTX has an absorption band in UVA region similar to folic acid, the UVA-induced damage to biomacromolecules may participate in the phototoxicity of MTX. MTX and DHP, a decomposed product of MTX, induced base oxidation especially at underlined G in 5'-GG-3' and 5'-GGG-3' (5'-TGGG-3') sequences in double-stranded DNA (Figure 11) [29].

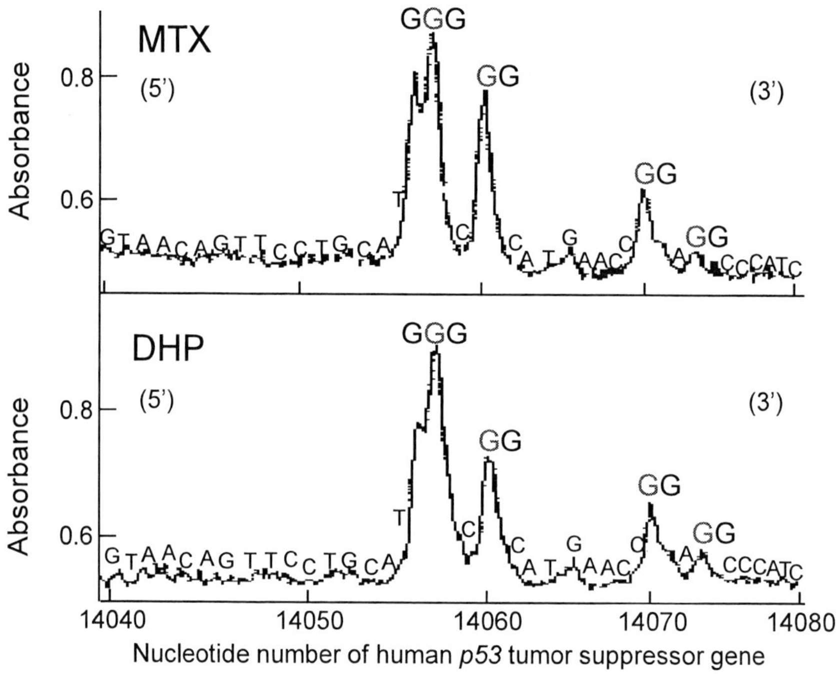

Figure 11. Sequence-specificity of DNA damage by photo-irradiated MTX and DHP.

This DNA cleavage pattern was quite similar to that by a type I photosensitizer, riboflavin [11,13,24]. The amount of 8-oxodGuo formation by photo-irradiated MTX in double-stranded DNA was much larger than that in single-stranded DNA. These results can be reasonably explained by assuming that nucleobase oxidation is induced by the activated photosensitizer mainly through electron transfer (type I mechanism) similar to the case of folic acid.

Formation of 8-oxodGuo by MTX or DHP increased depending on the photo-irradiation time. The 8-oxodGuo formation by DHP was significantly larger than that by MTX. An induction period (approximately 15 min) was observed in the 8-oxodGuo formation by MTX, suggesting that MTX itself could cause no or little DNA oxidation, and reactive species, unconjugated pteridines (UPT) including DHP, DFP, and DPC, generated from photo-irradiated MTX induced DNA oxidation. The 8-oxodGuo formation is roughly expressed as follows:

$$\mathrm{UPT} + h\nu \rightarrow \mathrm{UPT}^* \tag{1}$$

$$\mathrm{UPT}^* + \mathrm{G} \rightarrow \mathrm{G}^{\cdot+} \rightarrow \text{8-oxodGuo} \tag{2}$$

where UPT* represents photoexcited UPT including the singlet and triplet excited states. The rate equation can be practically expressed using the reaction rate constants, k_{ox1} and k_{ox2} as follows:

$$d[\mathrm{G}^{\cdot+}]/dt = k_{ox1}\,[\mathrm{UPT}^*][\mathrm{G}] = k_{ox1}\,\mathrm{I}\,[\mathrm{UPT}][\mathrm{G}] \tag{3}$$

$$d[\text{8-oxodGuo}]/dt = k_{ox2}[\mathrm{G}^{\cdot+}] \tag{4}$$

where [G], $[G^{\cdot+}]$, [8-oxodGuo], [UPT], and [UPT*] are concentrations of G, $G^{\cdot+}$, 8-oxodGuo, ground state of UPT, and UPT*, respectively. The nondimensional coefficient "I" depends on the number of photons absorbed by UPT. The analysis of the time course of 8-oxodGuo formation has been obtained by numerical calculation. On the basis of the assumption that photoexcited UPT generated from MTX oxidizes guanine, although photoexcited MTX does not, the time course of 8-oxodGuo formation was calculated by the equations (3) and (4) using above-mentioned k_{ox1} and k_{ox2}. This kinetic study demonstrated the idea that the DNA oxidation is due to UPT generated from MTX similar the DNA photodamage by folic acid. Folic acid analogues have pteridine ring, which is a potentially strong photosensitizer. Photodecomposition of these folic acid analogues may contribute to the photocarcinogenesis.

4. Application of Folic Acid Analogues: Fluorometry of ROS

4.1. Strategy for the ROS Detection

Folic acid consists of the base pteridine and *p*-aminobenzoyl-L-glutamic acid The calculated energy levels of the HOMO, the next HOMO, and the LUMO showed that the HOMO is located on the aminobenzoyl moiety of folic acid, suggesting that the fluorescence from the pteridine moiety can be quenched through intra-molecular electron transfer from the aminobenzoyl moiety [8]. It has been reported that the C_9-N_{10} bond connecting the pteridine and the aminobenzoyl moieties is unstable for oxidative stress [20,21]. ROS-mediated cleavage of this C_9-N_{10} bond should recover the fluorescence intensity of the pteridine moiety (Figure 12).

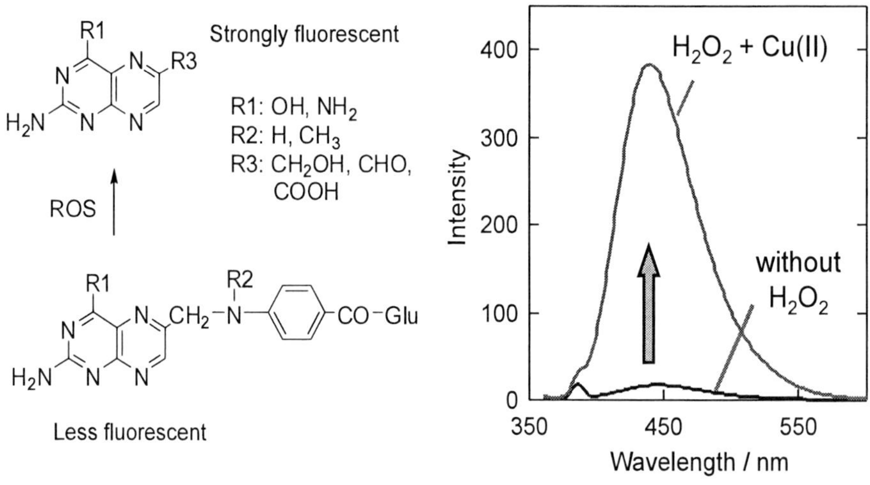

Figure 12. Fluorescence enhancement of folic acid analogue through the oxidative decomposition by H_2O_2 in the presence of copper(II) ion. The right spectra show the fluorescence enhancement of folic acid by H_2O_2 plus copper(II) ion.

These characters of folic acid analogues are advantageous for ROS detection. For example, the fluorescent method for determination of peroxynitrite using folic acid was reported [58]. These experiments were performed using barbital buffer solution and Hela cells, and it has been reported that the detection limit is 1.0×10^{-8} M in this solution.

4.2. Fluorometry of Hydrogen Peroxide

Hydrogen peroxide (H_2O_2) is one of the most important ROS. H_2O_2 plus Cu(II) markedly enhanced the fluorescence of folic acid and increased the fluorescence intensity in a dose-dependent manner, suggesting the decomposition of folic acid [16]. The shape of the fluorescence spectrum of the decomposed product of folic acid was quite similar to that of PCA. The decomposed products of folic acid were analyzed with an HPLC and demonstrated the idea that H_2O_2 induced the cleavage of the C_9-N_{10} bond of folic acid, resulting in the formation of PCA and *p*-aminobenzoyl-L-glutamic acid similar to the UVA reaction. At pH 7.6, folic acid exhibited optimum stability [6], and the sensitivity was independent on pH in the range 6.0 ~ 8.0. The limit of detection (LOD; at S/N=3) for H_2O_2 was 0.5 μM under this experimental condition. The fluorescence intensity of folic acid was not increased by H_2O_2 without the metal ion, indicating that H_2O_2 itself does not decompose folic acid. Two scavengers of •OH, ethanol and mannitol, showed an inhibitory effect on the decomposition of folic acid but could not completely inhibit the decomposition. H_2O_2 and Cu(II) are considered to generate other reactive species, including copper-peroxo intermediates, which are less reactive than •OH [13]. Relevantly, a reactive species generated from H_2O_2 and Cu(II) cannot be completely quenched by typical •OH scavengers but effectively damages biomacromolecules, such as DNA [13,59,60]. These findings demonstrate that folic acid can be selectively used for the fluorometry of H_2O_2 in the presence of Cu(II). In addition, the Cu(II)-mediated decomposition of folic acid by H_2O_2 proceeded linearly with the reaction time. The concentration of H_2O_2 can be determined by a calibration curve method.

4.3. Evaluation of Carcinogenic Compounds Using Folic Acid

The formation of a fluorescent molecule through the oxidative decomposition of folic acid is applicable to the detection of H_2O_2 and/or the evaluation of oxidative stress, namely, the biomolecular-damaging activities of compounds via H_2O_2 generation.

The activity of carcinogenic semicarbazide ($NH_2NHCONH_2$), which can damage DNA through the formation of H_2O_2 during the autooxidation process (Figure 13) [61], was examined. Semicarbazide induced the fluorescence enhancement of folic acid in the presence of Cu(II) [16]. This decomposition reaction was completely inhibited by catalase, indicating the involvement of

H_2O_2. This method could be applied to the detection of small amounts of H_2O_2 (LOD of generation rate; 0.01 μM min^{-1}) generated from a carcinogenic compound.

4.4. Fluorometry of Singlet Oxygen by Folic Acid Analogues

Singlet oxygen ($^1O_2$) is one of the most important ROS in the mechanism of the photosensitized oxidation of biomacromolecules [62-64]. The similar method of H_2O_2 detection using folic acid could be applied for the fluorometry of $^1O_2$. Folic acid and MTX were decomposed into a strongly fluorescent pteridine via a photosensitized reaction by methylene blue or other $^1O_2$-generating photosensitizers in a deuterium oxide solution (Figure 14) [17].

Sodium azide, a $^1O_2$ quencher, inhibited the fluorescence enhancement, indicating the contribution of $^1O_2$ to the decomposition of these folic acid analogues.

The contribution of $^1O_2$ to the fluorescence enhancement was estimated by subtracting the increased fluorescence of the sample with sodium azide from that without sodium azide. The resulting value of the fluorescence intensity increased in proportion to the irradiation time or the number of photons absorbed by the photosensitizer. The value of the enhanced fluorescence intensity per number of photons absorbed by the photosensitizer linearly increased with the $^1O_2$ quantum yield of the photosensitizers.

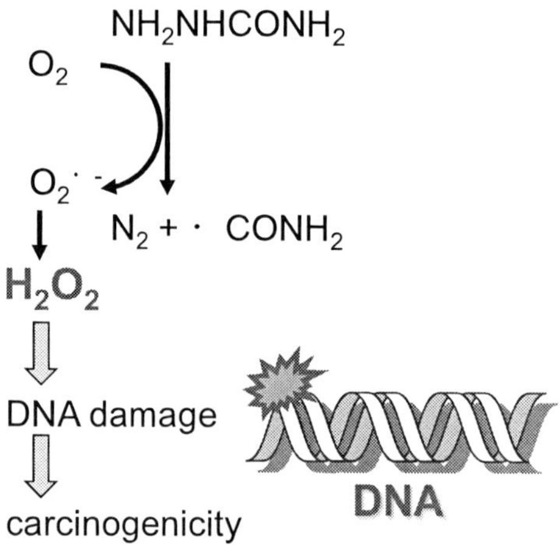

Figure 13. Autooxidation of semicarbazide and the generation of H_2O_2.

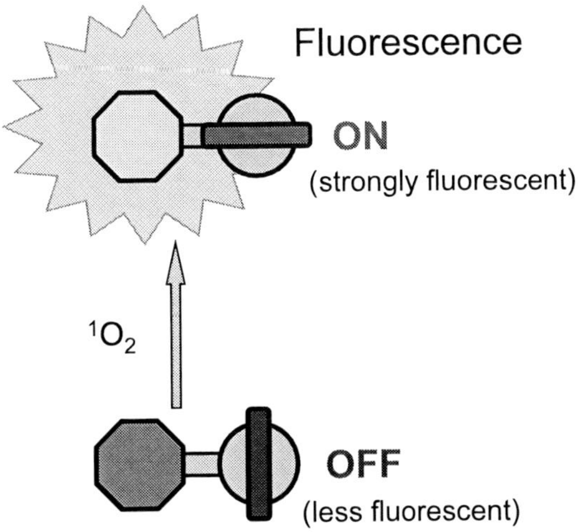

Figure 14. Scheme of the fluorescence enhancement of folic acid analogue by $^1O_2$.

This method using the fluorescence enhancement of these folic acid analogues can be applied to determine the quantum yield of $^1O_2$ generated through a photosensitized reaction in deuterium oxide. The roughly estimated reaction rate constant of MTX with $^1O_2$ was 3.1×10^6 M^{-1} s^{-1}, which is comparable to the previously reported value of folic acid [65]. The background fluorescence of MTX is quite smaller than that of folic acid, indicating that MTX can be used for the more sensitive detection of $^1O_2$.

Conclusion

Folic acid and MTX are decomposed into unconjugated pteridines by UVA irradiation, H_2O_2, and $^1O_2$ generated from photosensitized reaction. Since the unconjugated pteridine is a strong type I photosensitizer, degradation of folic acid in human skin may participate in solar-induced DNA damage, possibly resulting in the initiation process of skin cancer. On the other hand, an electron-donating aminobenzoyl moiety quenches the photoexcited pteridine of folic acid. It is speculated that the attachment with the aminobenzoyl moiety prevents the UVA-induced phototoxic effect by the pteridine moiety. The decomposition of folic acid and MTX markedly enhances their fluorescence intensity. These compounds can be used as fluorescence probe for ROS, including H_2O_2 and $^1O_2$ generated from photosensitized reaction.

References

[1] Young, K. J.; Lee, P. N. (1999). Statistics and computing Ltd, surrey, UK. Intervention studies on cancer. *Eur. J. Cancer Prev. 8*, 91-103.

[2] Giacosa, A.; Filiberti, R.; Hill, M. J.; Faivre, J. (1997). Vitamins and cancer chemioprevention. *Eur. J. Cancer Prev. 6*, S47-S54.

[3] Molloy, A. M.; Scott, J. M. (2001). Folates and prevention of disease. *Publ. Health Nutr. 4*, 601-609.

[4] Davis, R. E. (2002). Effects of folic acid. *Lancet 359*, 2038-2039.

[5] McCaddon, A.; Hudson, P.; Ellis, D.; Hill, D.; Lloyd, A. (2002). Effect of supplementation with folic-acid on relation between plasma homocysteine, folate, and vitamin B12. *Lancet 360*, 173.

[6] Akhtar, M. J.; Khan, M. A.; Ahmad, I. (1999). Photodegradation of folic acid in aqueous solution. *J. Pharm. Biomed. Anal. 19*, 269-275.

[7] Akhtar, M. J.; Khan, M. A.; Ahmad, I. (2003). Identification of photoproducts of folic acid and its degradation pathways in aqueous solution. *J. Pharm. Biomed. Anal. 31*, 579-588.

[8] Hirakawa, K.; Suzuki, H.; Oikawa, S.; Kawanishi, S. (2003). Sequence-specific DNA damage induced ultraviolet A-irradiated folic acid via its photolysis product. *Arch. Biochem. Biophys. 410*, 261-268.

[9] Off, M. K.; Steindal, A. E.; Porojnicu, A. C.; Juzeniene, A.; Vorobey, A.; Johnsson, A.; Moan, J. (2005). Ultraviolet photodegradation of folic acid. *J. Photochem. Photobiol. B: Biol. 80*, 47-55.

[10] Song, Q. –H.; Hwang, K. C. (2007). Direct observation for photophysical and photochemical processes of folic acid in DMSO solution. *J. Photochem. Photobiol. A: Chem. 185*, 51-56.

[11] Hiraku, Y.; Ito, K.; Hirakawa, K.; Kawanishi, S. (2007). Photosensitized DNA damage and its protection via a novel mechanism. *Photochem. Photobiol. 83*, 205-212.

[12] International Agency for Research on Cancer (IARC) Working Group, Solar and ultraviolet radiation, in: IARC Monographs on the Evaluation of Carcinogenic Risks to Humans, Vol. 55, IARC, Lyon, 1992, pp. 43-281.

[13] Kawanishi, S.; Hiraku, Y.; Oikawa, S. (2001). Sequence-specific DNA damage induced by UVA radiation in the presence of endogenous and exogenous photosensitizers. *Curr. Probl. Dermatol. 29*, 74-82.
[14] Kawanishi, S.; Hiraku, Y.; Oikawa, S. (2001). Mechanism of guanine-specific DNA damage by oxidative stress and its role in carcinogenesis and aging. *Mutat. Res. 488*, 65-76.
[15] Ito, K.; Kawanishi, S. (1997). Photoinduced hydroxylation of deoxyguanosine in DNA by pterins: sequence specificity and mechanism. *Biochemistry 361*, 774-781.
[16] Hirakawa, K. (2006). Fluorometry of hydrogen peroxide using oxidative decomposition of folic acid. *Anal. Bioanal. Chem. 386*, 244-248.
[17] Hirakawa, K. (2009). Fluorometry of singlet oxygen generated via a photosensitized reaction using folic acid and methotrexate. *Anal. Bioanal. Chem. 393*, 999-1005.
[18] Gomes, A.; Fernandes, E.; Lima, J. L. F. C. (2005). Fluorescence probes used for detection of reactive oxygen species. *J. Biochem. Biophys. Methods. 65*, 45-80.
[19] Thomas, A. H.; Lorente, C.; Capparelli, A. L.; Pokhrel, M. R.; Braun, A. M.; Oliveros, E. (2002). Fluorescence of pterin, 6-formylpterin, 6-carboxypterin and folic acid in aqueous solution: pH effects. *Photochem. Photobiol. Sci. 1*, 421-426.
[20] Taher, M. M.; Lakshmaiah, N. (1987). Hydroperoxide-dependent folic acid degradation by cytochrome c. *J. Inorg. Biochem. 31*, 133-141.
[21] Taher, M. M.; Lakshmaiah, N. (1987). Studies on hydroperoxide-dependent folic acid degradation by hemin. *Arch. Biochem. Biophys. 257*, 100-106.
[22] Patro, B. S.; Adhikari, S.; Mukherjee, T.; Chattopadhyay, S. (2005). Possible role of hydroxyl radicals in the oxidative degradation of folic acid. *Bioorg. Med. Chem. Lett. 15*, 67-71.
[23] Akhtar, M. J.; Khan, M. A.; Ahmad, I. (2000). Effect of riboflavin on the photolysis of folic acid in aqueous solution. *J. Pharm. Biomed. Anal. 23*, 1039-1044.
[24] Hirakawa, K.; Yoshida, M.; Oikawa, S.; Kawanishi, S. (2003). Base oxidation at 5' site of GG sequence in double-stranded DNA induced by UVA in the presence of xanthone analogues: relationship between the DNA-damaging abilities of photosensitizers and their HOMO energies. *Photochem. Photobiol. 77*, 349-355.

[25] Scurachio, R. S.; Skibsted, L. H.; Metzker, G.; Cardoso, D. R. (2011). Photodegradation of folate sensitized by riboflavin. *Photochem. Photobiol.87*, 840-845.

[26] Elisei, F.; Latterini, L.; Aloisi, G. G.; Mazzucato, U.; Viola, G.; Mioio, G.; Vedaldi, D.; Dall'Acqua, F. (2002). Excited-state properties and in vitro phototoxicity studies of three phenothiazine derivates. *Photochem. Photobiol. 75*, 11-21.

[27] International Agency for Research on Cancer (IARC) Working Group (1980) in IARC Monographs on the Evaluation of the Carcinogenic Risk of Chemicals to Humans, Vol 26, IARC, Lyon.

[28] Thaçi, D. (2008). Long-term data in the treatment of psoriasis. *Br. J. Dermatol. 159*, 18-24.

[29] Hirakawa, K.; Aoshima, M.; Hiraku, Y.; Kawanishi, S. (2002). Photohydrolysis of methotrexate produces pteridine, which induces poly-G-specific DNA damage through photoinduced electron transfer. *Photochem. Photobiol. 76,* 467-472.

[30] Chahidi, C.; Morliere, P.; Aubailly, M.; Dubertret, L.; Santus, R. (1983). Photosensitization by methotrexate photoproducts. *Photochem. Photobiol. 38*, 317-322.

[31] Chahidi, C.; Giraud, M.; Aubailly, M.; Valla, A.; Santus, R. (1986). 2,4-Diamino-6-pteridinecarboxaldehyde and an azobenzene derivative are produced by UV photodegradation of methotrexate. *Photochem. Photobiol. 44*, 231-233.

[32] Drobetsky, E. A.; Turcotte, J.; Chateauneuf, A. (1995). A role for ultraviolet A in solar mutagenesis. *Proc. Natl. Acad. Sci. USA 92*, 2350-2354.

[33] Besaratinia, A.; Synold, T. W.; Chen, H. H.; Chang, C.; Xi, B.; Riggs, A. D.; Pfeifer, G. P. (2005). *DNA lesions induced by UV A1 and B radiation in human cells: comparative analyses in the overall genome and in the p53 tumor suppressor gene. Proc. Natl. Acad. Sci. USA 102,* 10058-10063.

[34] Cohn, B. A. (2002). Sunlight, skin color, and folic acid. *J. Am. Acad. Dermatol. 46*, 317-318.

[35] David-Cordonnier, M. H.; Laval, J.; O'Neill, P. (2000). Clustered DNA damage, influence on damage excision by XRS5 nuclear extracts and Escherichia coli Nth and Fpg proteins. *J. Biol. Chem. 275*, 11865-11873.

[36] Burrows, C. J.; Muller, J. G.; (1998). Oxidative nucleobase modifications leading to strand scission. *Chem. Rev. 98*, 1109-1151.

[37] Lewis, F. D.; Wu, Y. (2001). Dynamics of superexchange photoinduced electron transfer in duplex DNA. *J. Photochem. Photobiol. C: Photochemistry Rev. 2*, 1-16.

[38] Steenken, S.; Jovanovic, S. (1997). How easily oxidizable is DNA? One-electron reduction potentials of adenosine and guanosine radicals in aqueous solution. *J. Am. Chem. Soc. 119*, 617-618.

[39] Sugiyama, H.; Saito, I. (1996). Theoretical studies of GG-specific photocleavage of DNA via electron transfer: significant lowering of ionization potential and 5'-localization of HOMO of stacked GG bases in B-form DNA. *J. Am. Chem. Soc. 118*, 7063-7068.

[40] Yoshioka, Y.; Kitagawa, Y.; Takano, Y.; Yamaguchi, K.; Nakamura, T.; Saito, I. (1999). Experimental and theoretical studies on the selectivity of GGG triplets toward one-electron oxidation in B-form DNA. *J. Am. Chem. Soc. 121*, 8712-8719.

[41] Ravanat, J. L.; Douki, T.; Cadet, J. (2001). Direct and indirect effects of UV radiation on DNA and its components. *J. Photochem. Photobiol. B: Biol. 63*, 88-102.

[42] Kasai, H.; Yamaizumi, Z.; Berger, M.; Cadet, J. (1992). Photosensitized formation of 7,8-dihydro-8-oxo-2'-deoxyguanosine (8-hydroxy-2'-deoxyguanosine) in DNA by riboflavin: a nonsinglet oxygen-mediated reaction. *J. Am. Chem. Soc. 114,* 9692-9694.

[43] Yamamoto, F.; Nishimura, S.; Kasai, H. (1992). Photosensitized formation of 8 -hydroxydeoxyguanosine in cellular DNA by riboflavin. *Biochem. Biophys. Res. Commun. 187*, 809-813.

[44] Cullis, P. M.; Malone, M. E.; Merson-Davies, L. A. (1996). Guanine radical cations are precursors of 7,8-dihydro-8-oxo-2'-deoxyguanosine but are not precursors of immediate strand breaks in DNA. *J. Am. Chem. Soc. 118,* 2775-2788.

[45] Spassky, A.; Angelov, D. (1997). Influence of local helical conformation on the guanine modifications generated from one electron DNA oxidation. *Biochemistry 36*, 6571-6576.

[46] Kino, K.; Saito, I.; Sugiyama H. (1998). Product analysis of GG-specific photooxidation of DNA via electron transfer: 2-aminoimidazolone as a major guanine oxidation product. *J. Am. Chem. Soc. 120*, 7373-7374.

[47] Kino, K.; Sugiyama, H. (2001). Possible cause of GC→CG transversion mutation by guanine oxidation product, imidazolone. *Chem. Biol. 8,* 369-378.

[48] Luo, W.; Muller, J. G.; Burrows, C. J. (2001). The pH-dependent role of superoxide in riboflavin-catalyzed photooxidation of 8-oxo-7,8-dihydroguanosine. *Org. Lett. 3*, 2801-2804.

[49] Bruner, S. D.; Norman, D. P. G.; Verdine, G. L. (2000). Structural basis for recognition and repair of the endogenous mutagen 8-oxoguanine in DNA. *Nature 403*, 859-866.

[50] Shibutani, S.; Takeshita, M.; Grollman, A. P. (1991). Insertion of specific bases during DNA synthesis past the oxidation-damaged base 8-oxodG. *Nature 349*, 431-434.

[51] McBride, T. J.; Schneider, J. E.; Floyd, R. A.; Loeb, L. A. (1992). Mutations induced by methylene blue plus light in single-stranded M13mp2. *Proc. Natl. Acad. Sci. USA 89*, 6866-6870.

[52] Negishi, K.; Hao, W. (1992). Spectrum of mutations in single-stranded DNA phage M13mp2 exposed to sunlight: predominance of G-to-C transversion. *Carcinogenesis 13*, 1615-1618.

[53] Sage, E.; Lamolet, B.; Brulay, E.; Moustacchi, E.; Chteauneuf, A.; Drobetsky, E. A. (1996). Mutagenic specificity of solar UV light in nucleotide excision repair-deficient rodent cells. *Proc Natl. Acad. Sci. USA 93*, 176-180.

[54] Okamoto, H.; Fukuda, A.; Mizuno, K.; Matsuyoshi, N.; Fujii, K.; Imamura, S. (1994). Reactivation of phototoxicity test for psoralens plus ultraviolet A by low-dose methotrexate. *Photodermatol. Photoimmunol. Photomed. 10*, 134-136.

[55] Morison, W. L.; Momtaz, K.; Parrish, J. A.; Fitzpatrick, T. B. (1982). Combined methotrexate-PUVA therapy in the treatment of psoriasis. *J. Am. Acad. Dermatol. 6*, 46-51.

[56] Andersen, K. E.; Lindskov, R. (1984). Recall of UVB-induced erythema in breast cancer patient receiving multiple drug chemotherapy. *Photodermatol. 1*, 129-132.

[57] Morison, W. L.; Marwaha, S.; Beck, L. (1997). PUVA-induced phototoxicity: incidence and causes. *J. Am. Acad. Dermatol. 36*, 183-185.

[58] Huang, J. -C.; Li, D. -J.; Diao, J. -C.; Hou, J.; Yuan, J. -L.; Zou, G. -L. (2007). A novel fluorescent method for determination of peroxynitrite using folic acid as a probe. *Talanta 72*, 1283-1287.

[59] Hirakawa, K.; Mori, M.; Yoshida, M.; Oikawa, S.; Kawanishi, S. (2004). Photo-irradiate titanium dioxide catalyzes site specific DNA damage via generation of hydrogen peroxide. *Free Radic. Res. 38*, 439-447.

[60] Hirakawa, K.; Oikawa, S.; Hiraku, Y.; Hirosawa, I.; Kawanishi, S. (2002). Catechol and hydroquinone have different redox properties responsible for their differential DNA-damaging ability. *Chem. Res. Toxicol. 15*, 76-82.

[61] Hirakawa, K.; Midorikawa, K.; Oikawa, S.; Kawanishi, S. (2003). Carcinogenic semicarbazide induces sequence-specific DNA damage through the generation of reactive oxygen species and the derived organic radicals. *Mutat. Res. 536*, 91-101.

[62] DeRosa, M. C.; Crutchley, R. J. (2002). Photosensitized singlet oxygen and its applications. *Coord. Chem. Rev. 233-234*, 351-371.

[63] Schweitzer, C.; Schmidt, R. (2003). Physical mechanisms of generation and deactivation of singlet oxygen. *Chem. Rev. 103*, 1685-1758.

[64] Hirakawa, K.; Hirano, T. (2008). The microenvironment of DNA switches the activity of singlet oxygen generation photosensitized by berberine and palmatine. *Photochem. Photobiol. 84,* 202-208.

[65] Cabrerizo, F. M.; Dántola, M. L.; Petroselli, G.; Capparelli, A. L.; Thomas, A. H.; Braun, A. M.; Lorente, C.; Oliveros, E. (2007). Reactivity of conjugated and unconjugated pterins with singlet oxygen ($O_2(^1\Delta_g)$): physical quenching and chemical reaction. *Photochem. Photobiol. 83*, 526-534.

In: Folic Acid
Editors: Mária Szabó and Eve Varga
ISBN: 978-1-62100-867-5

Chapter VIII

Folic Acid and B12 Supplementation Improves Survival of Elderly Hemodialysis Patients

Marco Righetti
Nephrology and Dialysis Unit, Cernusco S/N Hospital,
Cernusco S/N, Milan, Italy

Abstract

A large part of hemodialysis patients is over 65 years old. They often have vitamin B deficiency, hyperhomocysteinemia and high mortality rate. Recent meta-analysis have shown a significant decrease of cardiovascular disease in hyperhomocysteinemic end-stage renal disease patients treated with folic acid, but until now there are no data about the long-term effect of folic acid plus vitamin B12 on survival rate.

A long-term observational analysis was performed to assess the effects of vitamin B therapy on survival rate of incident hemodialysis patient over 65 years old. A large part of hemodialysis patients derived from previous prospective studies analysing the effects of folic acid on cardiovascular morbidity. 189 patients started haemodialysis, but only 141 patients had a follow-up time larger than 3 months. The mean age was 76 ± 0,5 years (65-86). The mean follow-up time was 959 ± 66 days (99-3518). 106 of 141 (75%) patients died. The median survival time was

2,7 years (0,3-9,6). Patients were sorted in two groups derived from folic acid and vitamin B12 treatment: group A (98 patients without vitamin B therapy or folic acid alone) and group B (43 patients with double vitamin B therapy). The median survival time was significantly different in the two groups: respectively equal to 1,8 years in group A and 3,9 years in group B (p< 0,01). Univariate regression analysis showed that death was directly dependent by age (χ^2: 8,2 ; p< 0,01), presence of central venous catheter at starting hemodialysis (χ^2: 10 – p< 0,01), late referral to our care (χ^2: 7 ; p< 0,01), and inversely related to double therapy with folic acid and vitamin B12 (χ^2: 18 ; p< 0,0001). Logistic multiple regression analysis demonstrated a strong reverse association between double vitamin B therapy and mortality (Coef/SE: -4,0 ; χ^2: 25,1 ; p value: <0,001).

Folic acid and vitamin B12 therapy was inversely associated with mortality in elderly hemodialysis patients. Homocysteine-lowering therapy may be useful to reduce cardiovascular and bone morbidity. Homocysteine-lowering effect may be reached with combination treatment using multivitamin B therapy, N-acetylcysteine and mixed dialysis therapies as high flux bicarbonate dialysis, internal hemodiafiltration, hemodiafiltration with endogenous reinfusion and on-line hemodiafiltration. Nowadays, it is important to perform a well-designed randomized controlled trial analyzing the effects of homocysteine-lowering therapies on hard end-points.

Keywords: Folic acid, vitamin B12, homocysteine, dialysis, cardiovascular disease, bone disease.

The Homocysteine-Lowering Folic Acid Effects on Cardiovascular Disease: A Never Ending Story

The overall mortality rate of hemodialysis patients is about 14% per year in Italy and cardiovascular mortality is actually responsible for about 40% [1]. Cardiovascular death is the most important cause of mortality both in the general population, and in patients with chronic renal failure [2,3]. Many studies have shown that high plasma homocysteine levels are responsible for 10% of the cardiovascular diseases and that homocysteine-lowering therapy, able to reduce total plasma homocysteine level of 5 micromoles/liter, lowers cardiovascular events rate of about 25% [4,5].

About 7 years ago a large observational study, the Dialysis Outcomes and Practice Pattern Study (DOPPS), detected an important association between the regular use of water-soluble vitamins, mainly folic acid, and the lower cardiovascular mortality rate of dialysis patients [6]. This study did not analyze the effects of vitamin B supplementation on homocysteine levels. At the same time, two interesting studies [7,8] showed that high plasma homocysteine levels were related to lower mortality rate of hemodialysis patients, hypothesizing an inverse epidemiology for total plasma homocysteine levels in patients with advanced chronic kidney disease. These two studies had really some methodological biases, because, first, either adjustment for malnutrition markers was not carried out or when it was performed the inverse association disappeared, and, second, diabetic patients on hemodialysis were a large part of the study population. My opinion is that it is important to analyze separately diabetic end-stage renal disease patients from the others one because they have at least two important confounding factors due to the diabetic disease: a high risk of cardiovascular morbidity typical of diabetic disease and total plasma homocysteine levels lower than non-diabetic ones with the same advanced chronic kidney disease [9]. The issue of reverse epidemiology between homocysteine and cardiovascular mortality in end-stage renal disease patients was not consequently established [10].

About 5 years ago my prospective study showed for the first time that homocysteine-lowering folic acid supplementation lowers cardiovascular morbidity of hemodialysis patients [11]. I also found both a positive association between homocysteine and supposed markers of nutritional status, as serum albumin and protein catabolic rate, and an inverse association between homocysteine and C-reactive protein, which is in agreement with a recent theory of a close relationship between malnutrition and inflammation. These last results were later confirmed [12]. Indeed, it was observed that the paradoxical reverse association between high total plasma homocysteine levels and lower mortality rate of dialysis patients may be due to the influence of wasting and inflammatory markers on plasma homocysteine levels. Therefore, all these results strongly support the theory that the influence of malnutrition and inflammation on homocysteine levels should be taken into consideration when evaluating homocysteine as a risk factor for cardiovascular morbidity and mortality of dialysis patients.

According to my data, supporting the protective effect of homocysteine-lowering folic acid therapy on cardiovascular events even though folic acid supplementation does not normalize plasma homocysteine levels in a large part of treated patients, it was observed [13] that long-term therapy with betaine, vitamin B and low-methionine diet is effective in lowering the cardiovascular mortality risk of patients with homocystinuria, a rare metabolic disorder, without reaching normal homocysteine values. Moreover, the effects of homocysteine-lowering folic acid supplementation on cardiovascular morbidity have been also analyzed in the population with small increase of total plasma homocysteine levels. It has been detected [14] that, after a food fortification program with folic acid, US and Canada population showed a highly significant decrease of fatal stroke as compared both with a similar population before the starting of this program and with the contemporary populations of England and Wales not submitted to a food fortification program with folate. The same differences observed with cerebrovascular events were achieved considering the effects of food fortification on neural tube defects. These data, even though the intervention model was not a randomized controlled trial which may represent the gold standard, were very important because they involved a large program of public health.

In 2006 a first meta-analysis [15], considering the effects of folic acid therapy on secondary prevention of cardiovascular events in randomized controlled trials, found no significant benefit or harm of folic acid treatment both on the risk of cardiovascular disease and all-cause mortality. Anyway it was observed, excluding VISP trial [16], a protective effect of folic acid supplementation on stroke (RR, 0.76; 95% CI, 0.63-0.93) and, consequently, the authors concluded that only other well-performed trials might provide a definitive answer to this important question of public health. VISP trial, although it showed that vitamin B therapy is ineffective to lower cardiovascular events rate, had two methodological biases: the absence of a placebo group and the presence of a food fortification program with folic acid which lowered homocysteine values in both patients' groups with, as result, a low difference for homocysteine levels in the two groups. Consequently, the authors tried to adjust their data analysis [17], showing that, if they chose two well-divided patients' subgroups for their vitamin B status, they noticed a significant risk reduction for composite cardiovascular events of patients treated with high doses of vitamin B and with high vitamin B12 levels.

In the same years the Norwegian Vitamin Trial (NORVIT) [18] published questionable results about homocysteine-lowering vitamin B effects on cardiovascular events because not only homocysteine values were similar in the treated and untreated groups, and these latter patients showed an unexpected increase of folate values during the study; but also plasma homocysteine levels were not an inclusion criteria, and thus a large part of enrolled patients had baseline total plasma homocysteine levels in the normal range or slightly increased. Hope-2 trial [19] was published with NORVIT in the same issue of the New England Journal of Medicine, and it was characterized by the same methodological biases. The baseline total plasma homocysteine levels were not an inclusion criteria, and consequently a large part of the enrolled study's population had not high homocysteine levels and folate deficiency because both they originated from fortification areas like US and Canada and they had taken vitamin B supplementation before starting the trial. Hope-2 trial told us that folic acid and vitamin B treatment does not reduce cardiovascular morbidity, but it was considered as unimportant the lower rate both of combined cardiovascular events (111 vs 147 cases, RR 0.76, 95% CI, 0.59-0.96, p= 0.03) and of non-fatal cerebrovascular events (84 vs 117 cases, RR 0.72, 95% CI, 0.54-0.95, p= 0.02) in the vitamin B subgroup as compared with the control group.

The randomized trials, excluding our study [11], showed a small decrease of plasma homocysteine levels from baseline that could signify a quite too short follow-up and, therefore, a weakness of the study to show the protective effect of homocysteine-lowering folic acid supplementation. The greatest effect of vitamin B therapy was surely achieved when this therapy was given to patients with high homocysteine levels, as early as possible, and for a long time. This theory was supported by a meta-analysis published on Lancet in 2007 [20]. The authors found, studying the efficacy of folic acid supplementation in the prevention of stroke, that folic acid treatment significantly lowered the risk of stroke by 18% (RR: 0.82, 95% CI: 0.68-1.00, p= 0.045) and this protective effect was detected in those studies with a long treatment, with a large homocysteine-lowering effect, in populations not submitted to fortified diets with folate, and in patients without previous history of stroke.

A recent meta-analysis [21] supported clear evidence that, on average, folic acid treatment may reduce cardiovascular disease risk in dialysis patients and in advanced chronic kidney disease patients by about 15%, and larger positive effect may be supposed in patients with sufficiently long period of therapy, in patients with larger decrease of homocysteine values during treatment, and in population without folic acid fortification.

This last meta-analysis, by pooling seven randomized trials (table 1) comprising a total of 3886 subjects with end-stage renal disease or advanced chronic kidney disease, achieved greater statistical power to reach a real conclusion. The sample size of the included trials varied, and the results were more likely influenced by the trials with larger sample size. However, the authors performed sensitivity testing and found that removing any single trial did not significantly change the positive results. They showed that, on average, folic acid treatment decreased the risk of cardiovascular disease by 15% in patients with end stage renal disease or advanced chronic kidney disease.

They observed, using a stratified analyses, a greater positive effect in the trials with a period of folic acid therapy longer than 24 months, with a decrease of homocysteine levels larger than 20%, and with no/partial grain fortification. The beneficial effect was also seen when the decrease of homocysteine levels was larger than 20% in the presence of folic acid fortification. It is important to notice that folic acid fortification of North Americans lowered the mean of homocysteine to about 8-10 micromoles per litre. It is probable that folic acid fortification might have contributed to the no-effect findings among these trials. This meta-analysis showed, as expected, that folic acid fortification was an important factor for the treatment effect of the trials [22,11,23,24,25,26,27]. To confirm the efficacy of folic acid therapy on cardiovascular disease in hyperhomocysteinemic patients with normal renal function, chronic renal failure or with end stage renal disease, future clinical studies should be performed in countries without folic acid fortification and in populations with low intake of folic acid, high homocysteine concentrations, and high frequency of cardiovascular disease.

Table 1. Table, adapted by Qin X et al (21), shows the most important trials considering the effects of homocysteine-lowering folic acid therapy on cardiovascular events

Data Source	Folate	Baseline hcy (μmol/L)	Δ hcy (%)	RR CVD
Righetti M et al [22]	5-15 mg/day	50,3	- 52,0	0,70
Righetti M et al [11]	5mg/day	35,0	- 40,6	0,73
Heinz J et al [23]	15 mg/week	29,0	- 30,0	0,84
Zoungas S et al [24]	15mg/day	27,0	- 17,4	0,85
Jamison RL et al [25]	40 mg/day	24,1	- 25,1	0,86
Vianna AC et al [26]	30 mg/week	25,0	- 55,3	0,87
Wrone E et al [27]	5-15mg/day	32,9	- 10,9	1,29

A significant risk reduction of cardiovascular disease was found in patients with high baseline homocysteine levels and a large homocysteine-lowering effect of folic acid therapy. Hcy: homocysteine; CVD: cardiovascular disease.

The first intervention trial with such patients' characteristics was designed [11] at the beginning of the third millennium. We performed this study in Italy, a country with no folic acid fortification, and we randomized 88 hemodialysis patients with low folate levels, hyperhomocysteinemia, exactly a mean value higher than 30 micromoles/litre, and a high cardiovascular events rate with more than 50% of the patients with previous cardiovascular events. Folic acid treated patients had a large decrease of total plasma homocysteine levels, about 15 micromole/litre starting from baseline plasma homocysteine values equal to 37,2 micromoles/litre, and a decrease of cardiovascular events rate equal to 27%. It is possible to postulate, considering our data, that 1 micromole/litre of homocysteine's decrease is associated to a reduction of cardiovascular events rate slightly lower than 2%. Also these last considerations may simply justify the unsuccessful results of the large randomized trials in patients with normal or with a mild increase of homocysteine levels. It is necessary to create a proper design of the study for showing the homocysteine-lowering effects on cardiovascular events. I agree with the conclusions of the last meta-analysis by Qin X and colleagues [21] who suggest a sufficiently long period of homocysteine-lowering therapy in hyperhomocysteinemic patients with high cardiovascular morbidity risk.

Folic Acid Plus B12 Therapy to Decrease Morbidity and Mortality of Hyperhomocysteinemic Patients

A further suggestion for planning future prospective trials on the effects of homocysteine-lowering therapy on overall and cardiovascular mortality may be derived from this last long study on the treatment of hyperhomocysteinemic dialysis patients [28]. We performed a long-term, observational study to assess the effects of vitamin B therapy on overall survival rate of incident hemodialysis patients over 65 years old, representing the largest part of dialysis patients with hyperhomocysteinemia, vitamin B deficiency and high mortality rate. A large part of the dialysis patients enrolled in this study derived from our previous prospective randomized study. In the last 11 years, beginning from January 2000, 189 patients over 65 years started hemodialysis in our centre, but only 141 of 189 patients had a follow-up time larger than 3 months. 48 patients were consequently excluded for a brief follow-up, less than 3 months. Data, collected from a SQL database, were analysed with

SPSS. The mean age was 76 ± 0,5 years (65-86). The mean follow-up time was adequately long, about 3 years (959 ± 66 days). Hemodialysis patients, as expected, had a high mortality rate: 106 of 141 (75%) patients died. The median survival time was 2,7 years (0,3-9,6). We sorted hemodialysis patients in two groups, according to the vitamin B therapy: 98 patients without vitamin B therapy or supplementation of folic acid alone (group A) and 43 patients treated with double vitamin B therapy: folic acid and B12 (group B). The median survival time was significantly different in the two groups: respectively equal to 1,8 years in group A and 3,9 years in group B ($p< 0,01$). We performed univariate regression analysis which showed that overall death was directly dependent by age (χ^2: 8,2 ; $p< 0,01$), presence of central venous catheter at starting haemodialysis (χ^2: 10 ; $p< 0,01$), late referral to our care (χ^2: 7 ; $p< 0,01$), and inversely related to double therapy with folic acid and vitamin B12 (χ^2: 18 ; $p< 0,0001$). Logistic multiple regression analysis (table 2) disclosed a strong reverse association between double vitamin B therapy and mortality (Coef/SE: -4,0 ; χ^2: 25,1 ; $p <0,001$). These results strengthened the hypothesis that multivitamin B therapies may decrease overall and cardiovascular mortality rate of our oldest hyperhomocysteinemic patients.

Dialysis patients have also high risk of bone fractures. An observational study, the Dialysis Outcomes and Practice Patterns Study (DOPPS), specified a high rate of fractures in dialysis patients, exactly 2.5 per 100 patients years for any type of fractures and 1 per 100 patients years for new hip fractures [29] Homocysteine was not measured in this large study, but it is known that homocystinuric patients, an interesting human model of patients with severe hyperhomocysteinemia, have osteoporosis due to collagen cross-links deficiency, but unrelated to collagen synthesis. Homocysteine may cause fractures, affecting bone matrix independently by bone mineralization.

In 2004 the Framingham Osteoporosis Study [30] showed that old patients with high homocysteine levels had a larger risk of hip fractures than patients with low homocysteine values. In the same number of the New England Journal of Medicine another study, Rotterdam and LASA studies [31], showed a strong association between high homocysteine levels and the risk of hip fractures. These results were independent by bone mineral density and other likely risk factors for fracture. Furthermore, a randomized controlled trial [32] detected that homocysteine-lowering vitamin B therapy decreases the risk of fractures in hemiplegic stroke patients. A few years ago I performed a retrospective analysis [33,34] considering the effects of folic acid supplementation on bone and cardiovascular events in dialysis patients. Dialysis patients were split into three groups according to response to folic acid therapy: folic acid responder (low homocysteine level, high folic acid and B12 values), folic acid resistant (intermediate homocysteine level, high folic acid and low B12 values) and a control group (high homocysteine level and low folic acid and B12 values).

We detected not only an inverse relationship between bone-cardiovascular events and grade of response to folic acid supplementation, but also no fractures in the responsive subgroup. These interesting results should be naturally confirmed by a long well-designed prospective trial able to study the effects of vitamin B supplementation on bone fractures in vitamin B deficient, hyperhomocysteinemic patients with high risk of bone disease.

Table 2. Table shows the logistic multiple regression analysis which demonstrates a strong reverse association between double vitamin B therapy and mortality (Coef/SE: -4,0 ; χ^2: 25,1 ; p value: <0,001)

Significant variables	Coef.	Chi-square	p
Double vitamin B	- 4,0	25,1	< 0,001
Age	0,15	9,0	< 0,01
Comorbidities	0,8	5,4	< 0,05

There was also a positive association with age and comorbidities which were computed by these five diseases: diabetes, coronary artery disease, cerebrovascular disease, cancer and liver disease. Univariate regression analysis also showed that mortality was directly dependent by other two variables: presence of central venous catheter at starting hemodialysis (χ^2: 10 – p< 0,01) and late referral to our care (χ^2: 7 ; p< 0,01).

Folic Acid and other Therapies Able to Reduce High Homocysteine Levels

I have recently observed in a prospective trial that folic acid and B12 replete patients have a mild time-dependent increase of homocysteine values which is higher in low-flux bicarbonate dialysis treated patients as compared with those treated with internal hemodiafiltration. Moreover the homocysteine removal capacity was significantly higher in internal hemodiafiltration than low-flux bicarbonate dialysis [35]. It is known that plasma homocysteine levels may be partially lowered with dialysis treatment. Low-flux bicarbonate dialysis removes a small part, about 30-35%, of pre-dialysis plasma homocysteine levels and homocysteine reduction rate during low-flux hemodialysis is lower than that of small molecules, as urea and creatinine, due to its protein binding. Plasma homocysteine values do not rise for at least 8 hours after low-flux dialysis in contrast to plasma creatinine concentration [36], and plasma homocysteine concentrations have a post-dialysis slight decrease if you consider end-stage renal disease patients treated with high flux bicarbonate dialysis able to remove middle molecules [37]. This typical homocysteine curve is suitable with an interesting theory that high flux bicarbonate dialysis may remove uremic toxins with inhibitory activities against one or more enzymes of the remethylation and/or transsulfuration pathway. High-flux dialysis membrane should perform this removal with larger efficiency. High-flux membranes with high capacity to eliminate large uremic substances, but without excessive leakage of useful proteins such as albumin, show an intradialytic higher homocysteine-lowering rate, about 40-50% compared to 30% of low-flux membrane. Moreover, pre-dialysis total plasma homocysteine values are slightly, but not significantly, lower in hemodialysis patients treated with high-flux membranes as compared to patients submitted to low flux dialysers during a follow-up time of 3 months [38]. The high-flux advanced polysulphone dialysers with high clearance of larger uremic toxins, but non-albumin-leaking, do not improve homocysteine clearance compared to high-flux standard polysulphone membranes, confirming that the large part of uremic toxins affecting homocysteine metabolism are protein-bound or have a molecular weight above 15000 Daltons [39]. The super-flux dialysers, albumin-leaking, improve pre-dialysis total plasma homocysteine values as compared to both low and high-flux membranes, by removing mainly large molecular weight solutes able to affect the homocysteine metabolism [40,41,42]

Some years ago I and my co-workers showed in a preliminary study that HFR, a special type of hemodiafiltration with endogenous reinfusion, and internal hemodiafiltration had high homocysteine-lowering effect [43] similar to super-flux membranes. It has been also observed that end-stage renal disease patients treated with on-line hemofiltration [44], nocturnal hemodialysis six or seven nights per week [45], and peritoneal dialysis [46,47] have significantly lower pre-dialysis total plasma homocysteine levels as compared to patients submitted to low-flux bicarbonate dialysis, probably because the first one removes larger molecular weight solutes and the others have a shorter inter-dialytic period which permits a less restricted diet. Indeed, total plasma homocysteine levels are not efficiently decreased by peritoneal dialysis because its dialytic removal via the peritoneal membrane is inefficient owing to its high protein-bound fraction [48] and, therefore, the reason of lower total plasma homocysteine levels in patients on peritoneal dialysis as compared to patients on standard hemodialysis is in theory due to the continuous treatment which gives the chance to the patients having a diet with more fruits and vegetables.

Vitamin B therapy represents actually the most important strategy to reduce homocysteine values. Serum folate levels have a high inverse association with plasma homocysteine concentrations. Folic acid supplementation normalizes total plasma homocysteine values in patients with normal renal function [49], but it is rarely able to control plasma homocysteine levels in patients with advanced chronic kidney disease. Some years ago I and my co-workers detected [22] that not only 15 mg oral daily folic acid supplementation was not better than 5 mg per day in lowering total plasma homocysteine values, but also that a large part, about 90%, of dialysis patients submitted to folic acid therapy had total plasma homocysteine values higher than the upper normal limit. It has been also observed that both higher doses of folic acid supplementation, equal to 30 or 60 mg per day, are not more useful than 5 mg per day in lowering plasma homocysteine levels [50], and betaine, added to folic acid, does not give additional homocysteine-lowering effect [51] indicative of a betaine-dependent remethylation not stimulated by exogenous betaine when patients are just treated with folic acid. Moreover, the homocysteine-lowering effect of intravenous folinic acid, oral folinic acid and oral folic acid is similar [52], suggesting that high homocysteine levels are not only due to abnormal folate metabolism.

In the following years I showed [47] that vitamin B therapy (5 mg oral daily folic acid, 1 mg intramuscular weekly vitamin B12 and 300 mg oral daily vitamin B6) largely improves total plasma homocysteine values, obtaining normal values in more than 70% of peritoneal dialysis patients. These clinical results are justified by the fact that methylation of homocysteine to methionine through the remethylation process needs vitamin B12 as enzymatic cofactor and transsulfuration of homocysteine to cystathionine through the transsulfuration process needs vitamin B6 as enzymatic cofactor. The literature's data suggest that there are no known severe side effects concerning folic acid treatment. The upper level of 1 mg oral daily folic acid of recommended dose [53] is due to the possible risk of masking anaemia in occasion of B12 deficiency. There are no known side effects also for vitamin B12 therapy, and apparently neither upper limits of intake. Vitamin B6 is important to reduce high total plasma homocysteine levels when added to vitamin B12 and folate, but single high doses of vitamin B6 are unsuccessful to lower hyperhomocysteinemia. Moreover, there is a safe upper limit for long-term vitamin B6 supplementation that is equal to 50-100 mg per day [53].

Table 3. Table shows the most important studies considering different strategies for lowering homocysteine levels in dialysis patients. iHDF: internal hemodiafiltration; BD: bicarbonate dialysis; HD: hemodialysis; hcy: homocysteine; HFR: hemodiafiltration with endogenous reinfusion; NAC: N-acetylcysteine

Data Source	Active treatment	Results
Righetti M et al [35]	iHDF vs. low-flux BD	iHDF is better than low-flux BD to remove hcy
House AA et al [38]	High-flux BD vs. low-flux BD	High-flux BD is better than low-flux BD to remove hcy
Van Telligen A [40]	Super-flux vs. high-flux vs low-flux	Super-flux is better than high-flux and low-flux to remove hcy
Righetti M et al [43]	HFR vs. low-flux BD	HFR is better than low-flux BD to remove hcy
Beerenhout C et al [44]	OL-HDF vs. low-flux BD	OL-HDF is better than low-flux BD to remove hcy
Friedmann AN et al [45]	Every day nocturnal HD vs. thrice weekly HD	Every day HD is better than thrice weekly HD to remove hcy
Moustapha A et al [46]	Peritoneal dialysis vs. low-flux BD	Peritoneal dialysis is better than low-flux BD to remove hcy
Righetti M et al [22]	5 mg vs. 15 mg oral daily folic acid	No differences for homocysteine-lowering effect
Sunder-Plassmann G et al [50]	5 mg vs. 30-60 mg oral daily folic acid	No differences for homocysteine-lowering effect
Van Guldener C et al [51]	Betaine in folic acid treated patients	No adding results for homocysteine-lowering effect
Ducloux D et al [52]	intravenous folinic acid vs. oral folinic acid vs. oral folic	No differences for homocysteine-lowering effect
Righetti M et al [47]	B6 plus B12 plus folic acid	Triple therapy is better than folic acid alone or double therapy (folic acid plus B12)
Thaha M et al [55]	Intravenous NAC during dialysis	Intravenous NAC during HD is better than HD without NAC

Moreover, end-stage renal disease patients treated with intravenous N-acetylcysteine showed lower post-dialysis plasma homocysteine values and better pulse pressure values as compared with untreated haemodialysis ones

[54,55]. It has been shown not only that patients submitted to 5 g intravenous acetylcysteine in 5% glucose solution for 4 hours during a single dialysis session had total plasma homocysteine levels clearly reduced (about 90%, with post-dialysis homocysteine values equal to 2 micromoles/liter) beyond the effects of hemodialysis treatment alone, but also that patients had an improvement of endothelial function. Intravenous acetylcysteine probably causes a fast displacement of homocysteine from protein-binding sites, allowing an increased rate of homocysteine available for clearance by hemodialysis, considering its small molecular weight. On the contrary, oral administration of acetylcysteine showed only a 20% of homocysteine-lowering as compared with the placebo group [56]. Unfortunately, a randomized controlled trial [57] showing a significant improvement of cardiovascular end-points in dialysis patients treated with acetylcysteine, 600 mg BID orally, did not evaluate the effects on homocysteine. Table 3 summarizes the know-how about the strategies to reduce homocysteine levels in renal disease patients.

Conclusion

This paper analyses the data of the last decade about the effects of homocysteine-lowering vitamin B therapy on bone and cardiovascular morbidity. It seems that homocysteine lowering strategies are useful to reduce morbidity and mortality rate of advanced chronic kidney disease/end-stage renal disease patients with moderate/severe hyperhomocysteinemia. It is important to confirm this strong suggestion with a well-designed randomized controlled trial.

References

[1] de Jager DJ, Grootendorst DC, Jager KJ, van Dijk PC, Tomas LM, Ansell D, Collart F, Finne P, Heaf JG, De Meester J, Wetzels JF, Rosendaal FR, Dekker FW. Cardiovascular and non cardiovascular mortality among patients starting dialysis. *JAMA*. 2009 Oct 28;302(16):1782-9.

[2] Baigent C, Burbury K, Wheeler D. Premature cardiovascular disease in chronic renal failure. *Lancet* 2000, 356: 147–52.

[3] Eknoyan G, Lameire N, Barsoum R, Eckardt KU, Levin A, Levin N, Locatelli F, MacLeod A, Vanholder R, Walker R, Wang H. The burden of kidney disease: improving global outcomes. *Kidney Int* 2004, 66: 1310–4.

[4] Graham IM, Daly LE, Refsum HM, Robinson K, Brattstrom LE, Ueland PM, Palma-Reis RJ, Boers GH. Plasma homocysteine as a risk factor for vascular disease. The European Concerted Action Project. *J. Am. Med. Assoc.* 1997, 277: 1775-81.

[5] Wald DS, Law M, Morris JK. Homocysteine and cardiovascular disease: evidence on causality from a meta-analysis. *Br. Med. J.* 2002, 325: 1202-8.

[6] Fissell RB, Bragg-Gresham JL, Gillespie BW, Goodkin DA, Bommer J, Saito A, Akiba T, Port FK, Young EW. International variation in vitamin prescription and association with mortality in the Dialysis Outcomes and Practice Patterns Study (DOPPS). *Am. J. Kidney Dis.* 2004, 44: 293-9.

[7] Kalantar-Zadeh K, Block G, Humphreys MH, Mcallister CJ, Kopple JD. A low, rather than a high, total plasma homocysteine is an indicator of poor outcome in hemodialysis patients. *J. Am. Soc. Nephrol.* 2004, 15: 442-53.

[8] Wrone EM, Hornberger JM, Zehnder JL, Mccann LM, Coplon NS, Fortmann SP. Randomized trial of folic acid for prevention of cardiovascular events in end-stage renal disease. *J. Am. Soc. Nephrol* 2004, 15: 420–6.

[9] Oishi K, Nagake Y, Yamasaki H, Fukuda S, Ichikawa H, Ota K, Makino H. The significance of serum homocysteine levels in diabetic patients on hemodialysis. *Nephrol Dial Tranplant* 2000; 15: 851-5.

[10] Ducloux D, Klein A, Kazory A, Devillard N, Chalopin JM. Impact of malnutrition-inflammation on the association between homocysteine and mortality. *Kidney Int* 2006, 69: 331-5.

[11] Righetti M, Serbelloni P, Milani S, Ferrario GM. Homocysteine-lowering vitamin B treatment decreases cardiovascular events in hemodialysis patients. *Blood Purif* 2006, 24: 379-86.

[12] Suliman M, Stenvinkel P, Qureshi AR, Kalantar-Zadeh K, Barany P, Heimbürger O, Vonesh EF, Lindholm B. The reverse epidemiology of plasma total homocysteine as a mortality risk factor is related to the impact of wasting and inflammation. *Nephrol Dial Transplant* 2007, 22: 209-17.

[13] Yap S, Boers GHJ, Wilcken B, Wilcken DEL, Brenton DP, Lee PJ, Walter JH, Howard PM, Naughten ER. *Arterioscler Thromb. Vasc. Biol.* 2001, 21: 2080-5.

[14] Yang Q, Botto LD, Erickson JD, Berry RJ, Sambell C, Johansen H, Friedman JM. Improvement in stroke mortality in Canada and the United States, 1990 to 2002. *Circulation* 2006, 13: 1335-43.

[15] Bazzano LA, Reynolds K, Holder KN, He Y. Effect of folic acid supplementation on risk of cardiovascular diseases. *JAMA* 2006, 296: 2720-6.

[16] Toole JF, Malinow MR, Chambless LE, Spence JD, Pettigrew LC, Howard VJ, Sides EG, Wang CH, Stampfer M. Lowering homocysteine in patients with ischemic stroke to prevent recurrent stroke, myocardial infarction, and death: the Vitamin Intervention for Stroke Prevention (VISP) randomized controlled trial. *JAMA* 2004, 291: 565-75.

[17] Spence JD, Bang H, Chambless LE, Stampfer MJ. Vitamin intervention for stroke prevention trial. An efficacy analysis. *Stroke* 2005, 36: 2404-9.

[18] Bønaa KH, Njølstad I, Ueland PM, Schirmer H, Tverdal A, Steigen T, Nordrehaug JE, Arnesen E, Rasmussen K, NORVIT Trial Investigators. Homocysteine lowering and cardiovascular events after acute myocardial infarction. *N. Engl. J. Med.* 2006, 354: 1578-88.

[19] Lonn E, Yusuf S, Arnold MJ, Sheridan P, Poque J, Micks M, McQueen MJ, Probstfield J, Fodor G, Held C, Genest J; Heart Outcomes Prevention Evaluation (HOPE) 2 Investigators. Homocysteine lowering with folic acid and B vitamins in vascular disease. *N. Engl. J. Med.* 2006, 354: 1567-77.

[20] Wang X, Qin X, Demirtas H, Li J, Mao G, Huo Y, Sun N, Liu L, Xu X. Efficacy of folic acid supplementation in stroke prevention: a meta-analysis. *Lancet* 2007, 369: 1876-82.

[21] Qin X, Huo Y, Langman CB, Hou F, Chen Y, Matossian D, Xu X, Wang X. Folic acid therapy and cardiovascular disease in end-stage renal disease and advanced chronic kidney disease: a meta-analysis. Clin *J. Am. Soc. Nephrol.* 2011; 6(3): 482-488.

[22] Righetti M, Ferrario GM, Milani S, Serbelloni P, La Rosa L, Uccellini M, Sessa A. Effects of folic acid treatment on homocysteine levels and vascular disease in hemodialysis patients. *Med. Sci. Monit.* 2003; 9: PI19-PI24.

[23] Heinz J, Kropf S, Domrose U, Westphal S, Borucki K, Luley C, Neumann KH, Dierkes J. B Vitamins and the risk of total mortality and

cardiovascular disease in end-stage renal disease: results of a randomized controlled trial. *Circulation* 2010; 121: 1432-1438.

[24] Zoungas S, McGrath BP, Branley P, Kerr PG, Muske C, Wolfe R, Atkins RC, Nicholls K, Fraenkel M, Hutchison BG, Walker R, McNeil JJ. Cardiovascular morbidity and mortality in the Atherosclerosis and Folic Acid Supplementation Trial (ASFAST) in chronic renal failure. *JACC* 2006, 47: 1108-16.

[25] Jamison RL, Hartigan P, Kaufman JS, Goldfarb DS, Warren SR, Guarino PD, Gaziano JM; Veterans Affairs Site Investigators. Effect of homocysteine lowering on mortality and vascular disease in advanced chronic kidney disease and end stage renal disease: a randomized controlled trial. *JAMA* 2007; 298: 1163-1170.

[26] Vianna AC, Mocelin AJ, Matsuo T, Morais-Filho D, Largura A, Delfino VA, Soares AE, Matni AM. Uremic hyperhomocysteinemia: a randomized trial of folate treatment for the prevention of cardiovascular events. *Hemodial. Int.* 2007; 11: 210-216.

[27] Wrone EM, Hornberger JM, Zehnder JL, McCann LM, Coplon NS, Fortmann SP. Randomized trial of folic acid for prevention of cardiovascular events in end stage renal disease. *J. Am. Soc. Nephrol* 2004; 15: 420-426.

[28] Righetti M, Ferrario G, Serbelloni P, Milani S, Tommasi A. Associazione diretta tra l'uso di vitamine B e la sopravvivenza dei pazienti anziani in emodialisi. *Giornale Italiano di Nefrologia* 2010; 27 (S51): S33

[29] Jadoul M, Albert JM, Akiba T, Akizawa T, Arab L, Bragg-Gresham JL, Mason N, Prutz KG, Young EW, Pisoni RL. Incidence and risk factors for hip or other bone fractures among hemodialysis patients in the Dialysis Outcomes and Practice Patterns Study. *Kideny Int* 2006; 70 (7): 1358-1366.

[30] McLean RR, Jacques PF, Selhub J, Tucker KL, Samelson EJ, Broe KE, Hannan MT, Cupples LA, Kiel DP. Homocysteine as a predictive factor for hip fracture in older persons. *N. Engl. J. Med.* 2004; 350: 2042-2049.

[31] van Meurs JB, Dhonukshe-Rutten RA, Pluijm SM, van der Klift M, de Jonge R, Lindemans J, de Groot LC, Hofman A, Witteman JC, van Leeuwen JP, Breteler MM, Lips P, Pols HA, Uitterlinden AG. Homocysteine levels and the risk of osteoporotic fractures. *N. Engl. J. Med.* 2004; 350: 2033-2041.

[32] Sato Y, Honda Y, Iwamoto J, Kanoko T, Satoh K. Effect of folate and mecobalamin on hip fractures in patients with stroke: a randomized controlled trial. *JAMA* 2005; 293: 1082-1088.

[33] Righetti M, Ferrario G, Serbelloni P, Milani S, Dossi C, Tommasi A. High bone and cardiovascular morbidity in folate-resistant hemodialysis patients. *Nephrol Dial Transplant Plus* 2008; 1(S2): ii211 (MO002).

[34] Righetti M. Protective effect of vitamin B therapy on bone and cardiovascular disease. Recent Patents on Cardiovascular *Drug Discovery* 2009, 4: 37-44.

[35] Righetti M, Filiberti O, Ranghino A, G Ferrario, S Milani, P Serbelloni, GE Guida, A Tommasi. Internal haemodiafiltration vs. low-flux bicarbonate dialysis: results from a long term prospective study. Int J *Artif Organs* 2010 Nov; 33(11): 796-802.

[36] Arnadottir M, Berg AL, Hegbrant J, Hultberg B. Influence of haemodialysis on plasma total homocysteine concentration. *Nephrol. Dial Transplant* 1999, 14: 142-6.

[37] Arnadottir M, Wingren K, Hultberg B, Hegbrant J. The postdialytic rise in the plasma total homocysteine concentration is delayed. *Blood Purif* 2002, 20: 334-7.

[38] House AA, Wells GA, Donnelly JG, Nadler SP, Hèbert PC. Randomized trial of high-flux vs low-flux haemodialysis: effects on homocysteine and lipids. *Nephrol Dial Transplant* 2000, 15: 1029-34.

[39] Mudge DW, Rogers R, Hollett P, Law B, Reiger K, Petrie JJB, Price L, Johnson DW, Campbell SB, Isbel NM, Sullivan M, Hawley CM. Randomized trial of FX high flux vs standard high flux dialysis for homocysteine clearance. *Nephrol Dial Transplant* 2005, 20: 2178-85.

[40] Van Telligen A, Grooteman MP, Bartels PC, Van Limbeek J, Van Guldener C, Wee PM, Nube MJ. Long-term reduction of plasma homocysteine levels by super-flux dialysers in hemodialysis patients. *Kidney Int.* 2001, 59: 342-7.

[41] De Vriese AS, Langlois M, Bernard D, Geerolf I, Stevens L, Boelaert JR, Schurgers M, Matthys E. Effect of dialyser membrane pore size on plasma homocysteine levels in hemodialysis patients. *Nephrol. Dial Transplant* 2003, 18: 2596-600.

[42] Galli F, Benedetti S, Buoncristiani U, Piroddi M, Conte C, Canestrai F, Buoncristiani E, Floridi A. The effect of PMMA-based protein-leaking dialyzers on plasma homocysteine levels. *Kidney Int.* 2003, 64: 748-55.

[43] Righetti M, Ferrario GM, Serbelloni P, Milani M, Tommasi A. Homocysteine reduction rate in internal haemodiafiltration: a

comparison with other mixed dialysis therapies. *Nephrol. Dial Transplant* 2006, 21: 2034-5.

[44] Beerenhout C, Luik AJ, Jeuken-Mertens SGJ, Bekers O, Menheere P, Hover L, Klaassen L, van der Sande FM, Cheriex EC, Meert N, Leunissen KM, Kooman JP. Pre-dilution on-line haemofiltration vs low-flux haemodialysis: a randomised prospective study. *Nephrol. Dial. Transplant* 2005, 20: 1155-63.

[45] Friedman AN, Bostom AG, Levy AS, Rosenberg IH, Selhub J, Pierratos A. Plasma total homocysteine levels among patients undergoing nocturnal vs standard hemodialysis. *J. Am. Soc. Nephrol* 2002, 13: 265-8.

[46] Moustapha A, Gupta A, Robinson K, Arheart K, Jacobsen DW, Schreiber MJ, Dennis VW. Prevalence and determinants of hyperhomocysteinemia in hemodialysis and peritoneal dialysis. *Kidney Int.* 1999, 55: 1470-5.

[47] Righetti M, Tommasi A, Lagona C, La Rosa L, Uccellini M, Sessa A. Effective homocysteine-lowering vitamin B treatment in peritoneal dialysis patients. *Perit Dial Int* .2004, 24: 373-7.

[48] Johnson DW, Kay TD, Vesey DA, Isbel N, Campbell SB, Hawley CM. Peritoneal homocysteine clearance is inefficient in peritoneal dialysis patients. *Perit Dial Int.* 2000, 20: 766-71.

[49] Homocysteine Lowering Trialists Collaboration. Lowering blood homocysteine with folic acid based supplements: meta-analyses of randomised trials. *BMJ* 1998, 316: 894-8.

[50] Sunder-Plassmann G, Födinger M, Buchmayer H, Papagiannopoulos M, Wojcik J, Kletzmayr J, Enzenberger B, Janata O, Winkelmayer WC, Paul G, Auinger M, Barnas U, Hörl WH. Effect of high dose folic acid therapy on Hyperhomocysteinemia in hemodialysis patients: results of the Vienna Multicenter Study. *J. Am. Soc. Nephrol.* 2000, 11: 1106-16.

[51] Van Guldener C, Janssen MJFM, Lambert J, ter Wee PM, Jakobs C, Donker AJ, Stehouwer CD. No change in impaired endothelial function after long-term folic acid therapy of hyperhomocysteinemia in hemodialysis patients. *Nephrol Dial Transplant* 1998, 13: 106-12.

[52] Ducloux D, Aboubakr A, Motte G, Toubin G, Fournier V, Chalopin JM, Drueke T, Massy ZA. Hyperhomocysteinemia therapy in hemodialysis patients: folinic versus folic acid in combination with vitamin B6 and B12. *Nephrol. Dial Transplant* 2002, 17: 865-70.

[53] Institute of Medicine. Dietary reference intakes for thiamine, riboflavin, niacin, vitamin B6, folate, vitamin B12, pantothenic acid, biotin, and choline. Washington DC, National Academy Press 2000, 150-95.

[54] Scholze A, Rinder C, Beige J, Riezler R, Zidek W, Tepel M. Acetylcysteine reduces plasma homocysteine concentration and improves pulse pressure and endothelial function in patients with end-stage renal failure. *Circulation* 2004, 109: 369-74.

[55] Thaha M, Yogiantoro M, Tomino Y. Intravenous N-acetylcysteine during haemodialysis reduces the plasma concentration of homocysteine in patients with end-stage renal disease. *Clin. Drug Investig* 2006, 26: 195-202.

[56] Friedman AN, Bostom AG, Laliberty P, Selhub J, Shemin D. The effect of N-acetylcysteine on plasma total homocysteine levels in hemodialysis: a randomised, controlled study. *Am. J. Kidney Dis*. 2003, 41: 442-6.

[57] Tepel M, van der Giet M, Statz M, Jankowski J, Zidek W. The antioxidant acetylcysteine reduces cardiovascular events in patients with end-stage renal failure. *Circulation* 2003, 107: 992-5.

Index

A

B

C

D

E

F

G

H

I

J

K

L

N

O

P

S

V

W

Y

Z